Neurological Case Histories

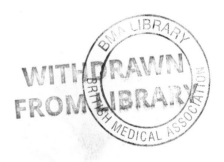

*This book has been printed digitally and produced in a standard specification
in order to ensure its continuing availability*

OXFORD
UNIVERSITY PRESS

Great Clarendon Street, Oxford OX2 6DP

Oxford University Press is a department of the University of Oxford.
It furthers the University's objective of excellence in research, scholarship,
and education by publishing worldwide in

Oxford New York

Auckland Cape Town Dar es Salaam Hong Kong Karachi
Kuala Lumpur Madrid Melbourne Mexico City Nairobi
New Delhi Shanghai Taipei Toronto
With offices in
Argentina Austria Brazil Chile Czech Republic France Greece
Guatemala Hungary Italy Japan South Korea Poland Portugal
Singapore Switzerland Thailand Turkey Ukraine Vietnam

Oxford is a registered trade mark of Oxford University Press
in the UK and in certain other countries

Published in the United States
by Oxford University Press Inc., New York

© Oxford University Press 2007

The moral rights of the author have been asserted

Database right Oxford University Press (maker)

Reprinted 2010

ISBN 978-0-19-263162-6

Neurological Case Histories

Case Histories in Acute Neurology and the Neurology of General Medicine

Sarah T Pendlebury
Honorary Consultant Physician,
John Radcliffe Hospital, Oxford

Philip Anslow
Consultant Neuroradiologist,
Radcliffe Infirmary, Oxford

and

Peter M Rothwell
Professor of Clinical Neurology,
University of Oxford Honorary Consultant Neurologist,
Radcliffe Infirmary, Oxford

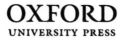

OXFORD
UNIVERSITY PRESS

Dedication

To our children, clinical colleagues, and patients.

Preface

The most interesting and challenging areas of medicine are often those where specialties overlap. In our opinion, emergency neurology and the neurology of general internal medicine, are among the most demanding areas of clinical practice, and are of particular importance in that many emergency and general medical neurological disorders are treatable. The differential diagnosis in such cases is often wide, but rapid diagnosis is of paramount importance since delay may cause significant harm.

Our aim in writing this book was to collect together a series of cases that would be of interest and educational value to physicians in general internal medicine, emergency medicine, and neurology. Most of the cases are either unusual presentations of common disorders or common presentations of rare but treatable conditions, with an emphasis on those that present acutely or which have a general medical component. It is no coincidence, therefore, that most of our cases first presented to emergency physicians or to general internal medicine physicians rather than directly to neurologists.

We chose the format of case reports with questions followed by answers including detailed discussions of the differential diagnosis and treatment for two reasons. First, because it is extremely difficult to illustrate the practical process of diagnosis within the traditional textbook format and, as in almost all areas of medicine, the best way to learn is through analysis of individual cases. Second, we believe it is simply more interesting to consider real cases and one's own differential diagnosis and treatment, than to read a text not requiring any effort on the part of the reader.

We would like to thank the following general physicians and neurologists for contributing cases and/or for helpful comments on the manuscript for this book: Professors Sir John Grimley Evans and Derek Jewell, and Drs Jane Adcock, Dennis Briley, Camilla Buckley, Ivor Byren, Jane Collier, Michael Donaghy, Richard Greenhall, Maggie Hammersley, David Hilton-Jones, Matthew Jackson, Bheeshma Rajagopolan, John Reynolds, Sudhir Singh, Simon Travis, Sunil Wimalaratna, and Simon Winner.

And especially to Dr Nicola Jones who contributed and commented on many of the infectious disease cases (and others).

Sarah Pendlebury, Philip Anslow, and Peter Rothwell

Contents

Symbols and abbreviations

↑	increased
↓	decreased
ABG	arterial blood gas
ADH	antidiuretic hormone (vasopressin)
AIDS	acquired immune deficiency syndrome
Alk phos	alkaline phosphatase
ANA	antinuclear antibody
ANCA	antineutrophil cytoplasmic antibody
AST	aspartate transaminase
Bili	bilirubin
BMI	body mass index
Ca	calcium
CMV	cytomegalovirus
CNS	central nervous system
CRP	c reactive protein
CSF	cerebrospinal fluid
CT	computed tomography
CXR	chest X-ray
EBV	Epstein–Barr virus
ECG	electrocardiogram
EEG	electroencephalogram
EMG	electromyogram
ENT	ear, nose, and throat
ESR	erythrocyte sedimantation rate
FBC	full blood count
FLAIR	fluid attenuated inversion recovery
FVC	forced vital capacity
GCS	Glasgow Coma Scale
GGT	gamma glutamyl transpeptidase
hep A,B	hepatitis A,B
HIV	human immunodeficiency virus
INR	international normalized ratio
ITU	intensive therapy unit
IVIG	intravenous immunoglobulin
LFT	liver function tests
LP	lumbar puncture
MMSE	mini mental state examination
MRI	magnetic resonance imaging
PCR	polymerase chain reaction
Plt	platelets
SAH	subarachnoid haemorrhage
SIADH	syndrome of inappropriate antidiuretic hormone (vasopressin) secretion
SLE	systemic lupus erythematosus
TB	tuberculosis
TFT	thyroid function tests
TIA	transient ischaemic attack
TSH	thyroid stimulating hormone
U&E	urea and electrolytes
WCC	white cell count

Normal ranges

Hb	13–18g/dL (men)
	11.5–16g/dL (women)
MCV	76–96fL
WCC	$4–11 \times 10^9$/L
Plt	$150–400 \times 10^9$/L
Na	135–145mmol/L
K	3.5–5mmol/L
Urea	2.5–6.7mmol/L
Cr	70–150µmol/L
Ca	2.12–2.65mmol/L
CK	25–195IU/L
CRP	<10mg/L
Glc (fasting)	3.5–5.5mmol/L
Bili	3–17µmol/L
AST	3–35IU/L
Alk phosp	30–300IU/L
GGT	11–51IU/L (men), 7–33IU/L (women)

Blood gases

PH	7.35–7.45
PaO_2	>10.6kPa
$PaCO_2$	4.7–6kPa
Bicarbonate	24–30mmol/L

CSF

Protein	0.15–0.45g/L
glc	2.8–4.2mmol/L
WCC	<5 lymphocytes/mm^3
Opening pressure	7–18cm H_2O

Case 1

A 29-year-old man presented with a 10-day history of sudden onset generalized headache and 2 days of depressed mood and apathy. There was no past medical history of note and he was not taking any medication. On examination, he was afebrile, the GCS was 15/15 and he was not confused (MMSE 30/30). General systems and neurological examination were unremarkable.

Investigations showed:

- Hb 13g/dL, WCC 13×10^9/L, platelets 200×10^9/L.
- CRP 30mg/L.
- U&E and LFT normal.
- CT brain: normal.
- LP: normal CSF opening pressure, protein 0.8g/L, cell count 15/mm^3 (12 mononuclear cells, 3 polymorphs), glucose 2mmol/L (blood glucose 5.6mmol/L), no organisms.

Over the course of the next day he became increasingly confused and the plantar responses became extensor. On examination, the temperature was 38.7°C, blood pressure 90/60 mmHg, he was intermittently unresponsive, restless, confused, and unable to follow commands, and there was a right-sided ptosis and bilateral extensor plantars.

An MRI scan was performed (see Fig. 1.1):

Questions

1a) Give the differential diagnosis you would have considered when the patient first presented, prior to the initial investigation results.

1b) Describe the findings on the MRI scan.

1c) What is the diagnosis and how would you confirm it?

1d) How would you treat this patient?

1e) What is the prognosis, and how has this changed over recent decades?

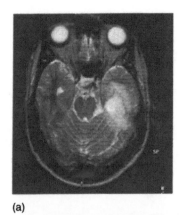

(a)

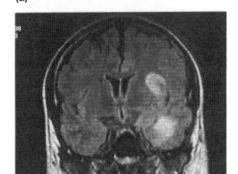

(b)

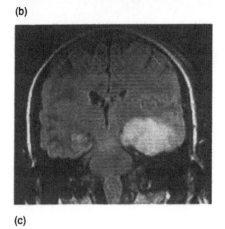

(c)

Fig. 1.1

Answers

1a) The differential diagnosis is for a subacute encephalopathy and includes:
- Infection:
  - TB, HSV, cryptococcus, toxoplasma, malaria, HIV, syphilis.
- Vascular disease:
  - CVT
  - Cerebral vasculitis.
- Neoplastic disorder.
- Other:
  - Depression
  - Hypothyroidism
  - CADASIL
  - MELAS
  - Hashimoto's encephalopathy
  - Drugs
  - Toxins e.g. mercury
  - Hepatic/renal failure.

The initial presenting features in this case were fairly non-specific and thus the differential diagnosis is wide. **Herpes simplex encephalitis** is probably the most likely cause since it produces behavioural change and headache and it is the most common cause of sporadic viral encephalitis in the industrialized world. Other viral agents should be considered in travellers and residents in other parts of the world. Non viral CNS infections that may present subacutely with altered mental state and headaches, particularly in immunosuppressed patients, are **toxoplasma gondii, crytococcus neoformans** (see page 42), and **TB** (see page 54). **Cerebral malaria, coccidioidomycosis,** and **blastomycosis** are possibilities in patients with recent travel to the Americas or Africa. A **space-occupying lesion** particularly of the frontal lobes should be considered in view of the personality change and headache. CNS infection is high on the list of differential diagnoses despite the absence of fever at the initial presentation.

CVT (see page 14) causes headache with or without reduced conscious level and focal neurological signs. Mitochondrial encephalopathy, lactic acidosis, and stroke-like episodes (**MELAS**) (see page 103) typically causes an encephalopathy, which may initially manifest as mood change, and focal neurological signs. **Hypothyroidism** causes depression and apathy and there are some reports of an association with headache. **Infiltrative disease of the CNS** e.g. leukaemia and lymphoma or malignant meningitis could cause headache and depression, likewise inflammatory CNS conditions such as **cerebral vasculitis** (see page 174) and **sarcoid** (see page 273). **Non-convulsive status epilepticus** (NCSE) typically causes behavioural change (see page 186) and headaches are common after seizure but in this case the headaches preceded the behavioural change. **Depression**, which is commonly associated with apathy, is associated with headache and other somatic complaints. **Illegal drug use** should be considered, particularly in younger patients where there is personality change.

1b) The MRI [axial T2-weighted MRI (Fig. 1.1a) and coronal FLAIR (Figs. 1.1b and 1c)] shows extensive oedema of the grey and white matter of the right insula and temporal lobe.

Asymmetrical temporal lobe abnormalities are often seen in herpes simplex encephalitis on MRI but CT (see Fig. 1.2) is less sensitive and is often normal early in the course of the disease. Temporal lobe changes are not exclusive to the diagnosis of herpes simplex encephalitis and extensive grey matter abnormalities may be seen with other encephalitides e.g. chicken pox (see Fig. 1.3). Temporal lobe change may also be seen in limbic encephalitis (see page 253).

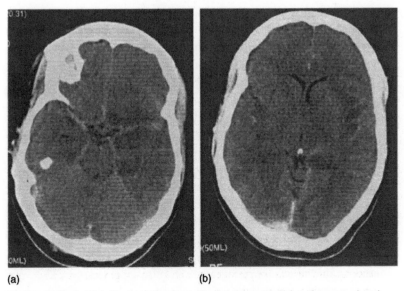

(a)   (b)

Fig. 1.2 CT brain showing hypodensity in the insular cortex (a) and temporal and inferior frontal lobes (b) in a patient with HSV encephalitis.

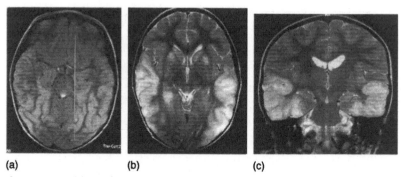

(a)   (b)   (c)

Fig. 1.3 FLAIR (a) and T2-weighted (b and c) MRI showing diffuse extensive bilateral grey matter hyperintensity in a child with chicken pox encephalitis.

1c) The diagnosis is **herpes simplex encephalitis.** PCR for herpes simplex virus (HSV) should be performed on the CSF. EEG may provide further supporting evidence.

The HSV virus invades the brain parenchyma and has a particular predilection for the temporal lobes, causing haemorrhagic necrosis. HSV-1 causes nearly all cases of HSV encephalitis in adults and oral herpes. HSV-2 causes genital disease, aseptic meningitis (see page 235), and congenitally acquired neonatal encephalitis. Both types have been associated with myelitis. There is no characteristic prodromal illness, or other clinical features that distinguish herpes simplex encephalitis from other causes of encephalitis. Fever, headache, confusion, bizarre behaviour, lethargy, stupor, seizures, hyperreflexia, and mild neck-stiffness are common. Hemiparesis (generally affecting the face and arm more than the leg), cranial nerve palsies, aphasia, and ataxia are less common. Superior quandrantanopias may occur. Infection and associated tissue injury predominantly involves the temporal and frontal brain regions and may be unilateral or bilateral. EEG may show seizure activity, sharp waves, and lateralized epileptiform discharges often localized to the frontotemporal regions. CSF shows a pleocytosis with lymphocytic predominance (5–500 cells/mm^3), moderately elevated protein (<1g/L) and normal or slightly low glucose.

In the past, brain biopsy was required to confirm the diagnosis of herpes simplex encephalitis, an invasive procedure associated with significant morbidity and mortality. More recently, PCR assay of CSF for the presence of DNA fragments to HSV has become the standard diagnostic test. In the first 4 days, PCR is positive in more than 95% of cases and remains so in 80% at one week. Although false positive tests do occur, this is limited to around 5% in most laboratories.

The EEG in herpes simplex encephalitis may show diffuse slowing, focal temporal region changes or periodic lateralized epileptiform discharge.

1d) Treatment is with intravenous aciclovir.

Intravenous aciclovir for 2–3 weeks should be given as soon as the diagnosis is suspected and before a definitive diagnosis is reached since early administration improves outcome (see below).

Renal function and hydration status should be monitored during treatment with aciclovir. Standard supportive therapy should be accompanied by antiepileptics if seizures occur. Use of steroids is controversial. Aciclovir resistant HSV has been described in immunocompromised patients for which foscarnet is the only treatment. Patients may relapse after completing therapy and biopsy may be necessary to distinguish ongoing viral infection from immune mediated disease.

1e) The use of aciclovir has greatly reduced the mortality from 70% prior to aciclovir use to 25–30%.

However, there is still significant morbidity and mortality associated with herpes simplex encephalitis. Persistent symptoms include memory impairment, poor concentration, irritability, emotional lability, and depression. Poor prognostic features include age over 30 years, presentation in coma, bilateral abnormalities on EEG, high CNS viral load, delayed treatment (4 days plus), and abnormal CT. The efficacy of steroids in herpes simplex encephalitis, principally for patients with increased intracranial pressure and oedema, has not been demonstrated in randomized trials.

Further reading

Cinque P, Cleator GM, Weber T, *et al*. (1996). The role of laboratory investigation in the diagnosis and management of patients with suspected herpes simplex encephalitis: a consensus report. *JNNP*; 61:339–345.

Hinson VK and Tyor WR (2001). Update on viral encephalitis. *Curr Opin Neurol*; 14:369–374.

Kennedy, PG (2004). Viral encephalitis: causes, differential diagnosis, and management. *J Neurol Neurosurg Psychiatry*; 75(1): 10–15.

McGrath N, Anderson NE, Croxson MC, Powell KF (1997). Herpes simplex encephalitis treated with acyclovir: diagnosis and long term outcome *J Neurol Neurosurg Psychiatry*; 63:321–326.

Raschilas F, Wolff M, DeIntour F, *et al*. (2002). Outcome of and prognostic factors for herpes simplex encephalitis in adult patients: results of a multicenter study. *Clin Infect Dis*; 35(3):254–260.

Case 2

Four case histories are described in brief below.

A) A 26-year-old pregnant woman presented with nausea, vomiting, and headache. There was no past medical history of note and she was not taking any medication. On examination she was drowsy and uncooperative but there was no focal neurology.

B) A 62-year-old woman presented with a 3-day history of generalized headache of gradual onset associated with neck stiffness and malaise. On the day of admission, she had awoken covered in blood with no memory of what had happened. She was taking tamoxifen for breast cancer diagnosed 6 months previously for which she had had a mastectomy. On examination, GCS was 14/15 and there was a laceration over the occiput. There was no focal neurological abnormality.

C) A 19-year-old woman presented with diarrhoea and vomiting, headache, and visual disturbance. She was a smoker and was taking the oral contraceptive pill. On examination, there was papilloedema and a right VI nerve palsy. She subsequently deteriorated developing bilaterally reduced visual acuity and bilateral VI nerve palsies and then right arm weakness.

D) A 31-year-old man presented with acute onset headache associated with right arm weakness. There was a past medical history of hepatic abscess and hepatic vein thrombosis. On examination, he was alert and there was no papilloedema but he had a right VI nerve palsy and right-sided pyramidal weakness. He had 2 generalized motor seizures in the emergency department.

Questions

2a) The diagnosis is the same in all 4 cases: what is it?

2b) What is the predisposing cause in each case?

2c) Give four other conditions associated with this diagnosis.

2d) How would you investigate these patients to confirm your diagnosis? Name one characteristic finding that is sometimes seen on brain imaging.

2e) What treatments may be given?

2f) What is the prognosis?

Answers

2a) The diagnosis is **cerebral venous sinus thrombosis (CVT).**

A schematic figure of the cerebral venous sinus system is shown in Fig. 2.1. In CVT, the superior sagittal sinus (see Figs. 2.2 and 2.3) and the transverse sinuses (see Figs. 2.3 and 2.4) are the most commonly affected followed by the straight sinuses (see Figs. 2.5 and 2.6) and the cavernous sinuses. More than one sinus is usually affected. Thrombosis of the Galenic system (see Fig. 2.6) or isolated involvement of the cortical veins is infrequent. CVT is often accompanied by raised intracranial pressure since the dural sinuses contain most of the arachnoid villi and granulations in which CSF absorption takes place.

Occlusion of one of the larger venous sinuses without involvement of cortical veins or the Galenic venous system generally causes raised intracranial pressure in the absence of focal neurological signs (apart

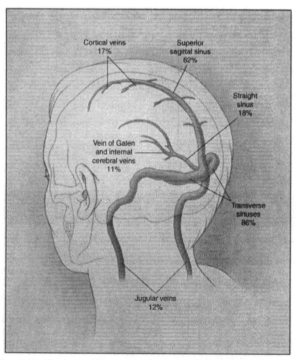

Fig. 2.1 Schematic diagram of the cerebral venous sinus system, reproduced with permission from Stam J (2005). Thrombosis of the cerebral veins and sinuses, *N Engl J Med.* **352**(17):1791–1798.

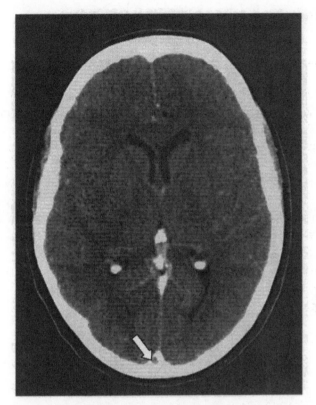

Fig. 2.2 CT brain with contrast from a young woman with sagittal sinus thrombosis who was taking the oral contraceptive pill. Arrow indicates the delta sign.

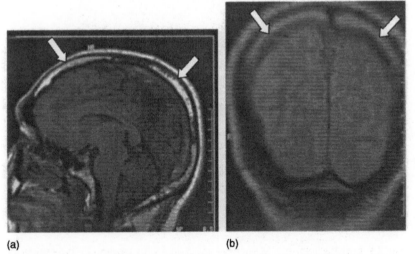

(a)   (b)

Fig. 2.3 Sagittal T1-weighted MRI (a) and proton density coronal MRI (b) showing hyperintensity in the region of the sagittal and transverse sinuses (arrows) respectively, consistent with thrombus.

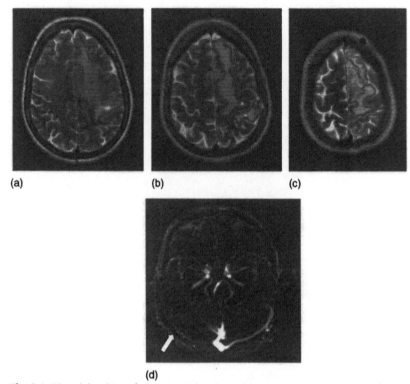

(a) (b) (c)

(d)

Fig. 2.4 T2-weighted MRI from case B showing white matter oedema in the left hemisphere (a,b,c) and thrombus (arrow) in the right transverse sinus on MRV (d).

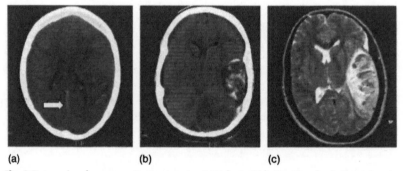

(a) (b) (c)

Fig. 2.5 Imaging from case D: Non contrast CT (a and b) showing fresh thrombus in the straight sinus (arrow) and haemorrhagic left temporal infarction shown also on T2-weighted MRI (c) performed subacutely when there was extensive oedema.

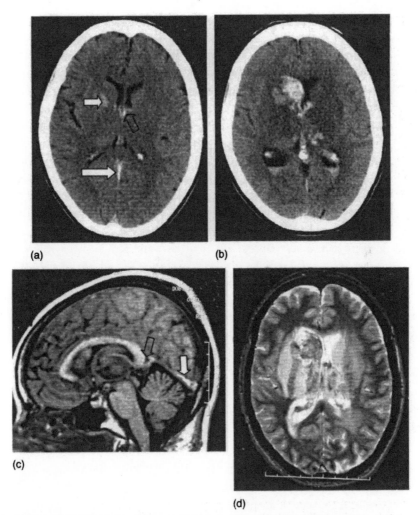

Fig. 2.6 Cerebral imaging from a patient presenting with headache, mutism, and depressed conscious level: Non contrast CT (a) showing fresh thrombus in the straight sinus (large arrow) and internal cerebral veins (open arrow) with early haemorrhagic infarct (small arrow). CT from the same patient 2 days later (b) shows extensive haemorrhagic infarction of the caudate nucleus and adjacent structures. MRI images are shown beneath for comparison: sagittal T1 image (c) showing fresh thrombus in the straight sinus (closed arrow), internal cerebral veins and veins of Galen (open arrow), axial T2-weighted image (d) showing massive haemorrhagic infarction of deep brain structures.

from VI nerve palsy occurring secondary to the raised pressure) since alternative drainage routes will be used. However, in cases of cortical vein involvement or extensive CVT, venous infarction, often accompanied by haemorrhage (around 40% at diagnosis), and subarachnoid bleeding (see page 141) may occur. Thrombosis of the straight sinus and Galenic system, which drain deep brain structures, may lead to bilateral thalamic infarction and akinetic mutism (see Fig. 2.6). Transient neurological deficits may be caused by temporary ischaemia and oedema.

The incidence of CVT is uncertain since it has a wide range of clinical manifestations and may be unrecognised or asymptomatic. The diagnosis should be suspected when a patient develops headache with or without focal neurological deficits, papilloedema and seizures, often with an apparently normal CT brain scan. Headache, which is often the presenting complaint, is present in 75–90% of cases and papilloedema occurs in about 50%. Focal deficits occur in around 30% and seizures in 40% (much higher than ischaemic stroke, see page 29). CVT should be considered in all cases of apparent benign intracranial hypertension (see page 220). Unusual presentations include psychosis, SAH (see page 141), cranial nerve disorders, TIA and migraine. Alternatively, symptoms may be obscured by the underlying disease process such as meningitis.

The progression of symptoms and signs in CVT is highly variable, ranging from less than 48 hours to greater than 30 days. A gradual onset over days or weeks of headache, papilloedema and less frequently VI nerve palsy, tinnitus and transient visual obscuration occurs in about 40% of cases.

2b) The predisposing cause is a prothrombotic tendency:

case A) pregnancy
case B) malignancy and tamoxifen
case C) smoking and the oral contraceptive pill
case D) previous hepatic vein thrombosis suggestive of a possible underlying procoagulant condition

2c) There are many conditions associated with CVTs of which the most important include pregnancy and the puerperium (5–20% and 25–60% of CVT in the developed and less developed world respectively), hormonal therapy, malignancy, dehydration, infection, and inflammatory disorders such as ulcerative colitis and Crohn's disease. In the past, otitis media was frequently complicated by transverse sinus thrombosis, so called 'otic hydrocephalus'. In the absence of other causes of CVT, hereditary coagulation disorders, for example factor V Leiden, should be carefully considered since they may require familial screening and probable long-term treatment.

2d) Investigations include:

- CT with contrast
- MRI and MRV
- Lumbar puncture.

Neuroimaging from cases B and D is shown in Figs. 2.4 and 2.5 respectively. CT with contrast (although normal in up to 25% of patients with proven CVT) would be an appropriate first line investigation particularly in sick patients in whom MRI can be difficult. Haemorrhagic and non-haemorrhagic infarcts, oedema and intense contrast enhancement of the falx and tentorium may be seen. Specific but less common changes include the 'delta sign' (see Fig. 2.2), a triangular pattern of enhancement from dilated venous collateral channels surrounding a central relatively hypodense area of thrombosis, indicating superior sagittal sinus thrombosis. Another is the 'cord sign' seen on a single slice only on non contrast enhanced CT scans in which fresh thrombus appears as increased density relative to grey matter in structures parallel to the scanning plane such as the straight sinus.

MRI has greater sensitivity than CT for the changes of CVT. In the acute phase (less than 3–5 days), the thrombus is isointense on both T1 and T2 sequences. Subsequently the thrombus becomes hyperintense. After 2–3 weeks, findings depend on whether or not the sinus remains occluded or whether it is partly or completely recannalised. Recently, MR angiography/venography (MRA/V) has enabled non-invasive visualization of the cerebral venous system. Catheter angiography is considered the gold standard for the diagnosis of CVT but nowadays should only be performed in those cases where the diagnosis remains in doubt after MRI.

The CSF is often abnormal in CVT: the pressure is frequently raised and there may be elevated protein and pleocytosis especially in patients with focal signs. Lumbar puncture may be indicated in patients with isolated intracranial hypertension to lower CSF pressure when vision is threatened and to exclude meningeal infection. EEG is abnormal in about 75% but changes are non-specific, with generalized slowing, often asymmetric, with superimposed epileptic activity.

2d) Treatment of CVT includes:

- Anticoagulation
- Treatment of raised intracranial pressure
- Anticonvulsants.

There is little evidence on the effectiveness of therapies for CVT although anticoagulants are widely used in the belief that they prevent extension of the clot into neighbouring sinuses and veins, which is often accompanied by rapid deterioration. Haemorrhage into a venous infarct is a recognized complication of anticoagulant therapy and since many patients recover spontaneously the risks may outweigh the benefits in some patients. However, since it is currently impossible to identify these patients, most clinicians advocate anticoagulant therapy in line with venous thromboembolism guidelines. Thrombolytic therapy, both via the intravenous and angiographic routes, has been used in patients with CVT but there is insufficient evidence to justify its use as a first line treatment. It should be reserved for patients who continue to deteriorate despite anticoagulation and supportive measures.

Intracranial hypertension resulting from CVT may cause death, seizures, visual failure, and focal deficits. Treatments include LP, steroids, mannitol, and acetazolamide. A minority of patients may require shunting. Anticonvulsants may be required for seizure prevention. Further therapies are aimed at the underlying cause of the CVT, e.g. infection or thrombophilia.

2e) The prognosis of CVT is very variable and difficult to predict for an individual patient: a comatose patient may go on to make a complete recovery whereas a patient with few signs may gradually deteriorate and die. The current case fatality appears to be 10–20% with 10–20% of surviving patients suffering persistent deficits.

Further reading

Bousser MG (2000). Cerebral venous thrombosis: diagnosis and management. *J Neurol;* 247(4):252–258. (Review.)

Ciccone A, Canhao P, Falcao F, Ferro JM, Sterzi R (2004). Thrombolysis for cerebral vein and dural sinus thrombosis. *Cochrane Database Syst Rev;* (1):CD003693.

Stam J. Thrombosis of the cerebral veins and sinuses (2005). *N Engl J Med;* 352(17):1791–1798. (Review.)

van Gijn J (2000). Cerebral venous thrombosis: pathogenesis, presentation and prognosis.*J R Soc Med;* 93(5):230–233.

Wasay M, Azeemuddin M (2005). Neuroimaging of cerebral venous thrombosis. *J Neuroimaging;* 15(2):118–128

Case 3

A 65-year-old gardener was brought by his wife to the outpatient clinic. She was concerned about his poor memory. He was able to give some details regarding his early life, although these were chronologically inaccurate, but he could remember nothing at all about the preceding 4 months. He was able to retain new information for a few minutes but then forgot it. His knowledge of current events was very poor.

Four months earlier, he had been admitted by the orthopaedic surgeons following a fractured elbow sustained when he had fallen downstairs. He was operated on later that day and 4 days after admission, he had been noted to be more confused and was thought to be hallucinating. On examination, absent ankle jerks and unsteady gait were found. The following day he had a seizure. His serum sodium was low at 125mm/L but normalized after fluid restriction.

Questions

3a) What is the diagnosis?

3b) Which conditions are associated with this diagnosis?

3c) What are the characteristic clinical features of this condition?

3d) What are the neuropathological changes?

3e) Could this patient's memory problems have been prevented?

Answers

3a) The diagnosis is Wernicke–Korsakoff syndrome.

3b) Conditions associated with Wernicke–Korsakoff syndrome include:

- Chronic alcoholism
- Hyperemesis gravidarum
- Anorexia nervosa
- Systemic malignancy
- Haemodialysis
- Gastrointestinal surgery
- Prolonged intravenous feeding
- Refeeding syndrome
- AIDS.

3c) Wernicke–Korsakoff syndrome is caused by thiamine (vitamin B1) deficiency.

Korsakoff syndrome is the chronic form of Wernicke–Korsakoff psychosis, the acute phase being Wernicke encephalopathy although since they represent two ends of a spectrum, symptoms and signs often overlap.

The patient described above developed Wernicke encephalopathy that was unrecognized during his surgical admission. It is often precipitated by metabolic stress such as severe infection, surgery or trauma, or a glucose or carbohydrate load. Wernicke encephalopathy is characterized by:

- Confusion, often with tremor and hallucinations or other features suggestive of delerium tremens
- Eye movement disorders: opthalmoplegia and nystagmus
- Truncal ataxia.

Abnormality of eye abduction is most common but any eye movement disorder can occur including internuclear opthalmoplegia and specific eye movement abnormalities may be difficult to identify. Pupillary abnormalities including sluggish reaction to light and near-light dissociation may be seen. The ataxia rarely affects the arms. Stupor and coma are rare. Hypothermia and postural hypotension may be present. Not all patients show these typical signs and this, together with the fact that not all patients admit to excess alcohol intake or may have other reasons for nutritional deficiency, means that many cases are unrecognized (only 20% in one case series).

Korsakoff syndrome is characterized primarily by profound memory impairment with other cognitive functions being relatively well preserved. The memory deficit is primarily anterograde i.e. there is an inability to acquire new information whilst more distant memories are retained, although not necessarily in chronological order. Retrograde amnesia is also seen. Most patients are disorientated in place and time. Confabulation may occur but is not pathognomic. Behavioural abnormalities include apathy, listlessness, and lack of insight. Examination findings include horizontal nystagmus, gait ataxia, and peripheral neuropathy.

Clinical evidence of thiamine deficiency in other systems includes oral or labial inflammation, peripheral oedema, and high output cardiac failure (e.g. beri beri). Signs of chronic liver disease may be present. Serum pyruvate may be elevated and thiamine-dependent erythrocyte enzyme transketolase activity is often reduced to half normal values. Enzyme activity may be restored by incubation with thiamine pyrophosphate (in practice these tests are not widely available and treatment is based on clinical suspicion).

3d) The neuropathological changes seen in Wernicke–Korsakoff syndrome are of necrosis and gliosis in the brainstem, hypothalamus, and thalamus.

The brainstem, thalamus, and hypothalamus are most affected, particularly the mamillary bodies, the walls of the third ventricle, the medial dorsal nucleus of the thalamus, the periaqueductal grey matter, the floor of the fourth ventricle, and the superior cerebellar vermis. Tissue necrosis affects neurons, axons and myelin. Glial proliferation occurs in more chronic lesions and is thus seen more in Korsakoff's syndrome than in Wernicke encephalopathy. Small haemorrhages may be seen. MRI may show shrunken mamillary bodies and CSF protein may be elevated.

The lesions in the medial dorsal and possibly the posterior nuclei of the thalamus are thought to be responsible for the memory impairment. Although cortical atrophy is seen in alcoholics, it is not thought that this is responsible for the typical cognitive changes seen in Korsakoff syndrome. Hypothalamic damage may rarely cause hypotension and hypothermia. Truncal ataxia is related to damage to the cerebellar vermis and eye movement abnormalities to lesions in the periaqueductal grey and pontine tegmentum (opthalomoplegias) and the vestibular complex at the pontomedullary junction (nystagmus).

3e) Wernicke encephalopathy should be treated with parenteral thiamine.

Wernicke encephalopathy is highly treatable and patients show improvement within hours of parenteral thiamine administration (the intravenous route should be used in the acute phase as oral absorption is unreliable). Untreated, there is a 10–20% mortality. Ocular palsies generally resolve completely within hours of treatment but there may be residual ataxia and horizontal nystagmus. Confusion or delerium resolves but patients may be left with memory impairment (Korsakoff syndrome) despite treatment. Thiamine should be given to any patient with unexplained stupor or coma. Administration of glucose may precipitate the acute Wernicke encephalopathy and thus thiamine should always be given together with glucose in hypoglycaemia if there is any suspicion of alcohol excess.

It is thought that immediate and aggressive treatment of Wernicke encephalopathy decreases the severity of subsequent Korsakoff syndrome. Treatment of established Korsakoff syndrome with regular thiamine may ameliorate memory dysfunction although improvement may take many months to appear and may not be maximal until at least 1 year.

Further reading

Cook CC, Hallwood PM, Thomson AD (1998). B Vitamin deficiency and neuropsychiatric syndromes in alcohol misuse. *Alcohol Alcohol*; 33(4):317–336.

Day E, Bentham P, Callaghan R, Kuruvilla T, George S (2004). Thiamine for Wernicke-Korsakoff Syndrome in people at risk from alcohol abuse. *Cochrane Database Syst Rev*; (1):CD004033.

Thomson AD (2000). Mechanisms of vitamin deficiency in chronic alcohol misusers and the development of the Wernicke–Korsakoff syndrome. *Alcohol Alcohol Suppl*; 35 Suppl 1:2–7.

Case 4

A 58-year-old retired female office clerk presented to the emergency services with dysphagia and leg weakness. Seven years previously, she had developed a cervical transverse myelitis which had resolved and then recurred 2 years later following which she was diagnosed with multiple sclerosis. Over the next 4 years she had several relapses that all presented with cord symptoms although brain MRI also showed demyelination. She had received treatment with interferon.

Three weeks prior to presentation, she was seen by her general practitioner with bilateral arm weakness and left leg weakness that had come on gradually over the previous 3 days. This was accompanied by tingling in the arms and legs that was possibly old. The general practitioner gave a 5-day course of prednisolone with initial improvement in her symptoms. One week before presentation, she developed dysphagia, nasal regurgitation, nasal voice and increasing limb weakness. There were no eye symptoms. Three days before, her face and upper limbs began to swell and the limb weakness worsened.

She was not on any medication. There was no family history or past medical history of note, she was an ex-smoker, and took minimal alcohol.

On examination, the arms and neck were oedematous and tender and the skin was flushed. There was mild lower limb oedema. General and breast examination was unremarkable. Her voice was weak with a poor cough. There was a left Horner's syndrome, weakness of eye closures and decreased palatal elevation. Swallow was impaired. Power was reduced proximally (severely in the lower limbs and moderately in the lower limbs) and to a lesser extent distally. Reflexes were absent in the upper limbs and ankles but present with reinforcement at the knees. Both plantars were upgoing. Vibration sense was reduced in both upper and lower limbs.

Questions

4a) What is the differential diagnosis? What do you think is the most likely diagnosis and why?

4b) Which other bedside test would you like to do?

4c) What other investigations would you request to confirm your diagnosis from 4a? What might you expect to find?

4d) In what percentage of patients with this condition is there an underlying disorder? What is the underlying disorder? Give 3 specific examples.

4e) How would you manage this patient?

Answers

4a) The differential diagnosis is:

- Acute myopathy e.g. dematomyositis (most likely diagnosis), rhabdomyolysis
- Acute neuropathy e.g. Guillain–Barré syndrome, porphyria
- Neuromuscular junction disorder e.g. myasthenia gravis.

This middle-aged woman presented with limb weakness, dysphagia with nasal regurgitation and swelling of the face and upper limbs on a background of multiple sclerosis. Examination showed predominantly proximal limb weakness with absent or reduced reflexes and upgoing plantars. When seen initially with limb weakness by the general practitioner, it was thought that she was experiencing a further attack of multiple sclerosis since all her previous relapses had been related to disease in the spinal cord. However, the subsequent findings of reduced or absent limb reflexes and symmetrical predominantly proximal upper and lower limb weakness do not fit with this diagnosis. Her existing demyelinating disease is likely to have been responsible for some of her symptoms and signs including the pins and needles in the limbs, Horner's syndrome, upgoing plantars and reduced vibration sense.

The pattern of predominantly proximal limb weakness developing over a 4-week period together with dysphagia, regurgitation and alteration in voice character is consistent with an acute myopathy. Although reflexes are usually preserved in myopathy, reduced or absent reflexes may be seen when the condition is particularly severe and in the current case, reflex elicitation may have been made more difficult by the presence of oedema. The relatively acute onset of symptoms, together with the accompanying flushed skin and oedema, makes dermatomyositis the most likely diagnosis.

Dermatomyositis is an inflammatory myopathy, affecting both children and adults with a female preponderance, in which there is a humoral autoimmune defect with complement mediated microangiopathy of muscle and skin. Presentation is acute or subacute over weeks or months. Skin manifestations with or without accompanying oedema may precede or accompany and an erythematous rash on the face, neck and anterior chest in a 'V' sign, or back, shoulders, knees, elbows and malleoli. A raised violaceous rash, Gottron's rash, at the knuckles and interphalangeal joints, is characteristic, as are dilated capillary loops at the base of fingernails. Calcium deposits in the skin are seen rarely in adults but when present they may extrude causing pain, ulceration and infection.

Limb weakness in dermatomyositis may be absent or severe and the extraocular muscles are never affected. Myalgia does not affect the majority of patients being present in only 30% of cases (in contrast to polymyalgia rheumatica in which pain rather than weakness is predominant). Bulbar and respiratory dysfunction may occur particularly in acute cases and cardiac abnormalities are seen including conduction defects and myocarditis. Pulmonary symptoms may occur secondary to muscle weakness or interstitial lung disease. Similar clinical features may be seen in myositis associated with scleroderma and other connective tissue diseases. The other acquired myopathies (see page 106 for a discussion) are generally insidious in onset although subacute presentation may occur in those caused by drugs/toxins, infection or critical illness. Involvement of the bulbar or respiratory muscles may occur in the latter.

Polymyositis is much rarer than dermatomyositis and is a disorder of cell mediated immunity in which cytotoxic T cells invade muscle fibres expressing MHC class 1 antigens leading to fibre necrosis. The skin is not affected. Polymyositis mimics many other myopathies and is a diagnosis of exclusion. It affects adults, being rare in children, and presents usually with insidious onset of proximal muscle weakness, although acute onset may occur. Bulbar dysfunction is rare and cardiac dysfunction does not occur. Many cases thought to be polymyositis in the past were probably inclusion body myositis (see below). Polymyositis is associated with a large number of autoimmune diseases, infections and inflammatory conditions including lupus, rheumatoid arthritis, HIV infection, sarcoid, primary biliary cirrhosis, and coeliac disease. It is also seen in association with D-penicillamine use in which case it responds to cessation of the drug. CK is always raised in active disease and EMG shows similar findings to those seen in dermatomyositis.

Inclusion body myositis is the most common inflammatory myopathy in men over the age of 50 years. There is early involvement of the quadriceps and long finger flexors, the latter being a strong pointer to the diagnosis. Involvement of the ankle dorsiflexors may occur leading to frequent falls. Progression is gradual but relentless and there is striking wasting of the distal muscles resembling a neuropathic picture and resulting in early impairment of fine finger movements in contrast to dermatomyositis and polymyositis in which such impairment is a late development. Dysphagia is common and rarely may be the presenting feature. Severe disability may result. Facial weakness is rare and muscle pain is usually absent. CK may be mildly elevated or normal.

The clinical syndrome of limb weakness, dysphagia and dysphonia with reduced or absent reflexes is typical of **Guillain–Barré syndrome** (see page 76). In Guillain–Barré syndrome, symptoms reach a maximum at 4 weeks, which is just within the period of illness described by this patient at presentation. In GBS, one might expect eye movement disorder to be present and more profound bilateral facial weakness. Limb weakness would not be predominantly proximal. There was no antecedent respiratory or GI upset recorded as is known to precede the development of GBS but this may not always be apparent. **Acute porphyria** may present with a similar clinical picture (page 65) but there were no other clinical features to suggest this diagnosis.

Myasthenic crisis may be the presenting form of myasthenia gravis in which there is bulbar dysfunction and ventilatory failure. However, ptosis and eye movement disorder are nearly always present, although purely proximal distribution of limb weakness may occur (limb girdle myasthenia), and reflexes are usually maintained.

Motor neuron disease causes bulbar symptoms, limb weakness and a mixture of upper and lower motor neuron signs. However, the development of symptoms is usually chronic. **Paraneoplastic** disorders include myopathy and neuropathy (see page 252) but the onset is usually insidious with relapsing and remitting features.

4b) The vital capacity should be measured and bulbar function monitored.

Patients with dermatomyositis may develop respiratory failure requiring ventilation and vital capacity should be monitored closely. It was 1.4L in this patient at the time she presented to the emergency physicians. Bulbar failure leading to airway compromise also indicates a need for intubation.

4c) Further investigations include:

- CK
- Inflammatory markers (often normal in dermatomyositis)
- Nerve conduction studies and EMG
- Muscle biopsy
- ECG.

In this patient, the CK was 6840IU/L with an AST of 281IU/L and LDH of 848IU/L. ESR was 92mm/h and CRP 42mg/L, albumin 24g/L. Elevation of CK to 50 times normal may be seen in dermatomyositis but levels may be normal even in active disease. Nerve conduction studies showed small sensory and motor responses with normal conduction velocity. Although a sensory motor axonal neuropathy could not be ruled out, it was felt that the small sensory and motor responses were likely to have been secondary to the presence of oedema. EMG showed acute denervation, increased spontaneous activity with fibrillations, positive sharp waves and a myopathic picture with small polyphasic motor unit action potentials. The combination of acute denervation and myopathic features on EMG is typical of an inflammatory myopathy (dermatomyositis, polymyositis and inclusion body myositis).

Muscle biopsy may be diagnostic of dermatomyositis (as it was in this patient) with perifascicular atrophy (a crust of small fibres surrounding a core of more normal sized fibres deeper in the fascicle) and prominent antibody labelling of MHC class 1 antigens. 'Ghost fibres', fibres undergoing degeneration and necrosis which have lost their staining characteristics, may be seen. Such diagnostic changes may not be seen in all patients with dermatomyositis and less specific inflammatory changes are seen. Skin biopsies show perivascular inflammation with CD4–positive cells in the dermis and dilated superficial capillaries in chronic disease. The histology is not distinguishable from cutaneous lupus.

In polymyositis, multifocal lymphocytic infiltrates surround the muscle fibres. Distinguishing polymyositis from other myopathies may be difficult. Muscle biopsy in inclusion body myositis shows cellular invasion of fibres, rimmed vacuoles and amyloid deposition and/or filamentous deposits.

Various antibodies e.g. anti-Jo-1, against nuclear or cytoplasmic antigens are found in around 20% of patients with inflammatory myopathies and are frequently associated with interstitial lung disease. They are not specific for disease subset and their role in the pathogensis of disease is unclear.

4d) Dermatomyositis is associated with underlying malignancy.

In the majority of patients with dematomyositis who have an underlying malignancy, the cancer is occult (the dermatomyositis is a paraneoplastic disorder (see page 252)). In one large study of 618 patients with dermatomyositis, 198 had cancer in which more than 50% were diagnosed after the dermatomyositis. Treatment of the underlying cancer usually improves the myopathy and relapse of cancer is associated with relapse of the myopathy. Many cancers have been reported to be associated with dermatomyositis including ovary, lung, pancreas, stomach, colon and rectum, and non-Hodgkins lymphoma. Childhood dermatomyositis does not appear to carry an increased cancer risk. There is a possible slight increase in cancer frequency in polymyositis.

4e) Treatment of severe acute dermatomyositis combines supportive measures including careful airway and swallow management with immunosuppression.

Steroids are the first line treatment and may be combined with other
immunosuppressants in severe disease or where steroid reduction causes
relapse. There is little trial evidence to guide therapy although azathio-
prine has been shown to be effective. Ciclosporin, mycophenolate mofetil
and methotrexate are also used. Double blind trials have shown effectiveness for IVIG but not plasma exchange. The CK level is a fairly good but
not infallible indicator of disease activity and treatment should be titrated
to improvement in weakness rather than to CK level. Older age and association with cancer are poor prognostic factors and morbidity is increased
in those with lung disease, frequent aspiration pneumonia secondary to
oesophageal dysfunction and calcinosis. Overall, at least a third of patients
are left with mild to severe disability.

Further reading

Callen JP (2001). Relation between dermatomyositis and polymyositis and cancer. *Lancet*;
357:85–86.

Dalakas MC and Hohlfeld (2003). Polymyositis and dermatomyositis. *Lancet*;
362(9388):971–982. Review.

Hilton-Jones D (2001). Inflammatory myopathies. *Curr Opin Neurol*; 14:591–596.

Case 5

A 78-year-old woman was admitted to hospital having had a tonic clonic seizure. She had been well until 3am on the day of admission, when she had woken up with a sensation of the room spinning. She had vomited and was unable to sit or stand, owing to unsteadiness. The unsteadiness and nausea resolved but she stayed in bed during the day. Her family called for an ambulance when she began to fit. There was no past medical history and she was on no medication.

On arrival of the admitting physician, tonic clonic movements had ceased and her GCS had increased from 8 to 14. She was apyrexial, with BM of 9.6mmol/L and BP of 186/92mmHg. There was no neck stiffness or photophobia but she continued to complain of feeling unsteady. She was leaning to the right in bed. There was mild dysarthria and nystagmus on right lateral gaze (fast component to the right) and right facial numbness. Tone, power and reflexes were normal and plantar reflexes were downgoing. Temperature and pin prick were reduced in the left upper limb.

Investigations showed:

- Hb 14.9g/dL, WCC 6.7 × 10^9/L, plt 197 × 10^9/L.
- Na 138mmol/L, K 3.8mmol/L, urea 4.5mmol/L, Cr 81μmol/L, chol 6.9mmol/L.
- ESR 15mm/h.
- ECG: normal axis, sinus rhythm.
- CXR: normal heart size, lungs clear.

Questions

5a) Where is the lesion?

5b) What are the two most likely diagnoses in order of preference and which other diagnosis would you have considered if she had been a young woman? What is the eponymous name given to the most likely diagnosis?

5c) What is the cause of this syndrome? What is the usual mode of onset?

5d) What other neurological symptoms and signs may occur in this syndrome?

5e) Are you surprised that this patient had a seizure given the most likely diagnosis? Would you prescribe an anti-convulsant?

5f) Which radiological tests would you request, and why?

Answers

5a) The lesion is in the brainstem (right side).

This patient presented with sudden onset of vomiting and vertigo and on admission was noted to have nystagmus on right lateral gaze, right limb ataxia and weakness, and left upper limb temperature and sensory loss. Vomiting and vertigo with nystagmus suggests a lesion of the vestibular apparatus, the vestibular nerve or its central connections in the brainstem. The presence of right-sided ataxia and left upper limb sensory loss indicate that the lesion is in the brainstem. Since the ipsilateral cerebellum controls coordination the lesion must be on the right. Pain and temperature sensation has been affected in the left upper limb as the pathways carrying this information through the medulla receive input from the contralateral limb (second order neurons cross to the contralateral side in the spinal cord at the level of the relevant peripheral neuron).

In this patient, the lesion was in the lateral medulla but inferior lateral pontine lesions may produce a similar clinical picture. Distinguishing between lateral medullary and pontine lesions may thus be difficult but the presence of ipsilateral palatal and vocal cord weakness (from involvement of the nucleus ambiguous) indicates the former and ipsilateral lower motor neuron facial weakness, VI nerve palsy and deafness indicates the latter.

5b) The two most likely diagnoses in order of preference are:

- **Lateral medullary infarction**
- Haemorrhage into a space occupying lesion.

Demyelination (MS) should be considered in younger patients with a brainstem syndrome.

Lateral medullary infarction is also known as **Wallenburg's syndrome**.

5c) The main arterial supply to the lateral medulla is from a number of penetrating arteries that originate from the distal vertebral artery (superior, middle or inferior lateral medullary arteries) and variably from small branches of the posterior inferior cerebellar, anterior inferior cerebellar and basilar arteries. Occlusion of any of these arteries may cause a lateral medullary infarct. Headache may occur in association with brainstem infarction but severe headache or neck pain, particularly if unilateral, should prompt investigation for dissection (see page 118).

The onset of lateral medullary infarction is sudden in only about 40% of cases. In the majority of patients, the course is gradual or stepwise over a

24–48 hour period. There is a preceding transient ischaemic attack with features of the lateral medullary syndrome in about 25% of patients as seen in the present case.

5d) Signs and symptoms that may be seen in Wallenburg's syndrome are shown below:

- Symptoms:
  - Ipsilateral facial sensory change
  - Vertigo
  - Nausea and vomiting
  - Ipsilateral clumsiness
  - Diplopia, oscillopsia
  - Numbness contralateral to the lesion
  - Dysphagia, hoarseness
  - Headache.
- Signs.
- Contralateral:
  - Impaired sensation over half the body, sometimes including the face.
- Ipsilateral:
  - Impaired facial sensation
  - Limb ataxia, falling to side of the lesion
  - Horner's syndrome
  - Dysphagia, hoarseness, vocal cord paralysis
  - Diminished gag reflex
  - Loss of taste.
- Other:
  - Nystagmus
  - Hiccup.

5e) A seizure in association with posterior circulation stroke is unusual.

Seizures are uncommon at onset of any type of stroke, occurring in about 5% of patients in the first week or two, usually in the first 24 hours and are more common in severe strokes, haemorrhagic stroke and those involving the cortex. The majority of seizures are partial with secondary generalisation. For all patients with stroke, there is a 3–5% risk of first seizure in the first year after stroke (excluding the first 2 weeks) falling to 1–2% a year thereafter. This represents a greatly increased seizure risk compared to that of the age–matched background population. The risk is lower in patients who become functionally independent and in those with posterior circulation or lacunar stroke.

It should be noted that post-seizure weakness (**Todd's paresis**) may mimic stroke in patients with other causes of seizure and non-convulsive status may cause aphasia of sudden onset that may be misdiagnosed as stroke (see page 187). Further, assessment of initial stroke severity is complicated in patients who have had a seizure at stroke onset as conscious level may be reduced and neurological deficits may be exacerbated. Finally, seizures at stroke onset may not necessarily be caused by the stroke itself and other causes of seizure should be excluded, including alcohol withdrawal, metabolic derangement, drugs, and hypertensive encephalopathy.

An isolated seizure following stroke does not usually warrant treatment unless the risk of recurrence is thought to be particularly high or unless the patient wishes to minimize the risk of further seizures because of the implications for driving restrictions, employment or leisure activities. There are no randomized trials comparing the different

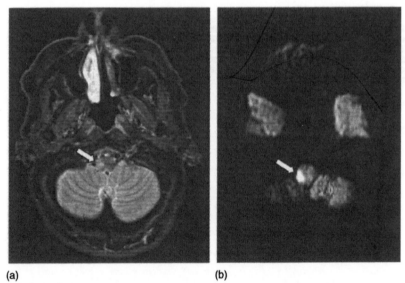

(a)　　　　　　　　　　　　　　(b)

Fig. 5.1 There is a T2-weighted hyperintensity in the right medulla (a) (arrow). On DWI, an axial slice at the same level (b) shows a hyperintense area (corresponding to the T2-weighted abnormality in the first image) consistent with an acute infarct.

anticonvulsants after stroke and phenytoin, valproate and carbamezepine are commonly used.

5f) Radiological tests include:

- CT brain (first line) to exclude haemorrhage
- MRI/MRA
- Conventional angiography if dissection suspected
- Diffusion weighted MRI (DWI).

CT brain would be the usual first line investigation as it will show any haemorrhage and may show a space-occupying lesion. MRI is more sensitive at showing brainstem lesions than CT and should be combined with MRA. The latter may show arterial dissection or occlusion in the posterior circulation. DWI is very sensitive for acute stroke which shows up as a strongly hyperintense area and is useful in differentiating acute from chronic infarction. The brain imaging from this patient is shown in Fig. 5.1.

Further reading

Burn J, Dennis M, Bamford J *et al* (1998). Epileptic seizures after a first-ever stroke: the Oxfordshire Community Stroke Project. *BMJ*; **315**:1582–1587.

Norrving B and Cronqvist S (1991). Lateral medullary infarction: prognosis in an unselected series. **41**:244–248.

Reith J, Jorgensen HS, Nakayama H *et al* (1997). Seizures in acute stroke: predictors and prognostic significance. The Copenhagen Stroke Study. *Stroke*; **28**:1585–1589.

Sacco RL, Freddo L, Bello JA (1993). Wallenburg's lateral medullary syndrome. Clinical-magnetic resonance imaging correlations. *Archives of Neurology*; **50**:609–614.

Case 6

An 80-year-old man was seen in the outpatient clinic with a 6-week history of falls and reduced mobility together with tingling in the feet, such that he was needing help to transfer and walk. He experienced mild pain in his hips and shoulders after trying to mobilize and said that his muscles 'felt stiff.' His wife reported that his memory had begun to deteriorate over the past year or so. There was a complicated past medical history including hypertension, which had proved difficult to control, ischaemic stroke, from which he had made a good recovery, and oesophageal cancer 5 years previously. He had also been admitted to the renal unit 7 months earlier with renal failure secondary to acute pyelonephritis and dehydration. His renal function had returned to normal on discharge. He was taking aspirin and antihypertensive medication (not β blockers). He lived with his wife and was an ex-smoker and drank moderate amounts of alcohol per week.

On examination, he was overweight with a pulse of 50/min and a blood pressure of 160/100. MMSE was reduced at 25/30 with deficits in recall and orientation. Cranial nerves were intact. There was normal tone in the limbs and no wasting. The upper limbs were moderately weak, more pronounced distally, and there was weakness of the lower limbs, predominantly of hip flexion and ankle dorsiflexion. Upper limb reflexes were intact but knee jerks were reduced and ankle jerks absent. Plantars were downgoing. Sensory examination revealed impaired vibration and joint position sense to the knee and reduced light touch in a glove and stocking distribution. There was no finger nose ataxia. He required help to get out of a chair and his gait was unsteady. Romberg's test was negative.

Investigations showed:

- Hb 10.4g/dL, MCV 89, WCC 4.0 × 10^9/L, plt 243 × 10^9/L, Na 133mmol/L, K 3.8mmol/L, Cr 123μmol/L, cholesterol 7mmol/L
- CXR: upper lobe blood diversion
- Nerve conduction studies: axonal and demyelinating sensorimotor peripheral neuropathy
- CT brain: evidence of an old right temporal stroke
- LP: protein 0.85g/L, no cells, glc normal.

Questions

6a) List the sites of lesion in the nervous system indicated by the history, examination and investigation results.

6b) What is the most likely diagnosis? What abnormalities might you see on laboratory investigation?

6c) Which alternative diagnoses would you have considered?

6d) Describe the neurological abnormalities associated with this condition.

Answers

6a) The clinical features of this case indicate:

- Diffuse cerebral dysfunction causing cognitive impairment
- Myopathy causing difficulty rising from a chair, proximal limb weakness and contributing to unsteady gait and difficulty mobilizing
- Sensorimotor neuropathy causing tingling in the feet, distal limb weakness and contributing to unsteady gait and difficulty mobilizing
- Previous right temporal stroke with good recovery.

6b) The most likely unifying diagnosis is **hypothyroidism**.

Hypothyroidism causes abnormalities in multiple sites of the nervous system (see below). This patient was found to have a grossly elevated TSH. Hypothyroidism is common in the elderly affecting up to to 14% of the elderly population and presentation may be non specific or atypical. Diagnosis is important as the condition is easily treated and neurological abnormalities are generally reversible. The cause is usually auto-immune gland destruction, post-radiation treatment for thyrotoxicosis, and thyroidectomy. Pituitary and hypothalamic disease are rare.

Metabolic changes in many organ systems cause numerous abnormalities on investigation. Diversion of blood away from the periphery to maintain body temperature causes diastolic hypertension (possibly accounting for the lack of response to treatment seen in this patient) and a decrease in blood volume. There is impairment of cardiac contractility and bradycardia that may cause congestive cardiac failure and CXR may show pleural and/or pericardial effusions. ECG shows bradycardia with low voltage complexes and prolongation of the QT interval. Reduction in free water clearance may result in hyponatraemia. Bone marrow function may be suppressed with a normocytic (usually although macrocytosis may occur) anaemia and impaired white cell response to infection. Decreased gluconeogenesis increases the likelihood of hypoglycaemia. Serum cholesterol may be elevated as well as the CK (see page 107) and LDH.

6c) Alternative diagnoses include:

- Giant cell arteritis/polymyalgia
- Alcohol excess
- B12 deficiency
- Paraneoplastic syndromes
- Inflammatory conditions
- Mitochondrial disease.

Giant cell arteritis commonly causes headache and constitutional symptoms including malaise, weight loss and fevers. However, it may present more insidiously. Stroke, and multi-infarct dementia have been reported as well as a peripheral neuropathy. There may be associated polymyalgia causing proximal weakness with moderate to severe pain in the limb girdle distribution.

Chronic alcohol abuse has wide effects on the nervous system and causes cognitive impairment often with pronounced memory impairment with confabulation (**Korsakoff's amnestic syndrome,** see page 18), a sensorimotor primarily axonal neuropathy with loss of vibration sense, and impaired reflexes and a myopathy. Cerebellar dysfunction may also occur.

B12 deficiency (see page 268) is common in the elderly and should be considered in any patient presenting with cognitive impairment and peripheral neuropathy. However, there are no features of myelopathy in this case and B12 deficiency is not associated with myopathy.

Paraneoplastic phenomena (see page 252) include cognitive impairment, neuropathy and myopathy but usually only one process is seen in any one patient. The mechanism is presumed to be antibody mediated and thus many of the specific syndromes e.g. limbic encephalitis are seen with specific cancers, in this case small cell lung cancer.

Sarcoid can cause encephalopathy, neuropathy, and myopathy (see pages 108 and 273). The encephalopathy can cause isolated memory impairment and strokes may occur secondary to vasculitis, compression from mass lesions or sarcoid-associated cardiomyopathy. Sensorimotor peripheral neuropathy (axonal) is the most common peripheral neuropathy. Myopathy may be acute or chronic and there may be associated muscle nodules. Other inflammatory conditions including rheumatological disorders may cause a similar picture (see page 288).

Mitochondrial disease e.g. MELAS (see page 103), can cause this combination of clinical features but there is nothing else clinically to suggest this diagnosis in this case.

6d) Multiple levels of the nervous system can be involved in adult hypothyroidism.

Abnormalities can be grouped into the following categories:

- Encephalopathy that may progress to seizures and coma
- Psychological changes especially depression
- Sleep disorders
- Cerebellar ataxia

- Cranial nerve lesions
- Myopathy
- Peripheral nerve disorders
- Other.

Slowness of thought, impairment of attention and concentration, somnolence and lethargy are common in hypothyroidism. Untreated patients may progress to myxoedema coma, usually occurring in elderly patients often after admission to hospital and precipitated by intercurrent illness. The cardinal features are coma with defective temperature control and a precipitating illness. Seizures occur in 20% and body temperature is low. There may be accompanying hypotension, respiratory failure and hypoglycaemia. There are no specific laboratory abnormalities other than those of hypothyroidism although this may mimic the sick euthyroid state and it may be necessary to measure free circulating hormone levels. CSF pressure is usually raised with an elevated protein. EEG is abnormal in myxoedema coma with a decrease in the frequency of alpha rhythm, reduction in photically evoked reposes, and an overall decrease in the amplitude and slowing of the dominant rhythm, often with low-range theta activity. Treatment of myxoedema coma includes intravenous thyroxine, hydrocortisone, broad spectrum antibiotics, correction of electrolyte abnormalities and respiratory and circulatory support.

Psychiatric features are common in hypothyroidism with depression being by far the most frequent manifestation. Thyroid function should always be checked in depressed patients especially where the patient is elderly. Significant cognitive impairment occurs in around a third of hypothyroid patients and may mimic dementia. Deficits in learning, memory, attention, verbal fluency and motor response times are seen. Rare psychiatric features of hypothyroidism include facetiousness suggestive of a frontal lobe disorder, irritability, paranoia, hallucinations, delirium, and psychosis (myxoedema madness). It is currently unclear whether cognitive deficits are fully reversible with thyroid hormone replacement: animal data suggest that there may be a therapeutic window within which full recovery is possible hence the importance of early diagnosis and treatment.

Sleep apnoea may occur in hypothyroidism. Obstructive sleep apnoea is caused in part by mucopolysaccharide deposition around the tissues of the upper airway cf mucopolysaccharide deposition causing carpal tunnel syndrome (see below). The cause of central sleep apnoea is unclear but reduced hypoxic drive and alterations in levels of CNS hormones may play a part.

Cerebellar dysfunction is common and associated symptoms may be the presenting feature of hypothyroidism: gait ataxia, impairment of balance and increased tendency to fall are particularly prominent. Such symptoms resolve rapidly with thyroid hormone replacement therapy. The pathophysiological basis for the cerebellar dysfunction is unclear but is assumed to be metabolic in origin.

Pituitary enlargement may occur in hypothyroidism owing to pituitary hyperplasia from lack of negative feedback on the pituitary from circulating thyroid hormones and this may cause subtle visual field defects through pressure on the optic chiasm. Hearing impairment and tinnitus are common and has conductive, neural and central components. Hoarseness of the voice is caused by structural changes in the vocal cords rather than neurological disease.

Muscle symptoms may be one of the first features of hypothyroidism but although elevation of CK occurs in the majority of hypothyroid patients, most patients are asymptomatic. Myopathy develops within a few weeks of biochemical hypothyroidism. Weakness, cramps, muscle aches and pains, particularly during and after exertion, slow movements and reflexes and affected muscles may be enlarged and have myoedema (transient local mounding when the muscle is percussed). Reflexes may be slow relaxing. EMG may show myopathic features. The painful stiff proximal muscles may lead to an incorrect diagnosis of polymyalgia. The weakness is usually mild and tends to affect the limb girdle preferentially but severe myopathy including rhabdomyolysis and respiratory insufficiency requiring ventilation have been reported. Diaphragmatic dysfunction may occur. Pathological changes in muscle are rather non specific and include atrophy, necrosis and hypertrophy of fibres, and increase in glycogen and connective tissue. Residual muscle weakness may persist despite treatment with thyroxine replacement therapy and many patients require months of treatment before improvement occurs.

Carpal tunnel syndrome is the most common peripheral nerve complication of hypothyroidism occurring in a significant minority of patients. Tarsal compression syndromes may also occur. Most patients do not require surgery since symptoms respond to treatment of the underlying disorder. One third of patients may have clinical evidence of a general polyneuropathy which is predominantly sensory with paraesthaesia, distal sensory loss, and impairment of distal joint position and vibration sense. Nerve conduction studies may show absent or decreased sensory nerve action potentials and slow motor conduction velocities consistent with either demyelination or axonal pathology. Pathological changes include demyelination and remyelination, axonal degeneration and increased glycogen and lysosomes in axonal and Schwann cell cytoplasm. Thyroid hormone replacement therapy usually improves the neuropathy.

Further reading

Duyff RF, Van den Bosch J, Laman DM *et al* (2000). Neuromuscular findings in thyroid dysfunction: a prospective and electrodiagnostic study. *JNNP*; **68**(6):750–755.

Osterweil D, Syndulko K, Cohen SN *et al* (1992). Cognitive function in non-demented older adults with hypothyroidism. *J Am Geriatr Soc*; **40**:325.

Case 7

A 20-year-old man presented to his GP with a 1-month history of gradual onset headache associated with malaise. The headaches were worse towards the end of the day and associated with photophobia. The GP found him to be thrombocytopaenic and referred him to a haematologist. On further questioning he had been nauseated for 2 weeks and had had blurred vision for 3 days. He had experienced blackouts over the preceding week. There were no witnesses to these episodes and he denied incontinence or tongue biting. He had felt non-specifically unwell for the preceding few months and had lost 10kg in weight. There was no past medical history other than a road traffic accident abroad 12 years previously in which he had sustained bilateral leg fractures and received a blood transfusion. He did not smoke or drink and worked as a car mechanic.

On examination, he was afebrile and had cervical lymphadenopathy and oral candidiasis. General systems were otherwise unremarkable. Examination of the nervous system revealed mild neck stiffness and photophobia, severe bilateral papilloedema, a right VI palsy and horizontal nystagmus most marked on looking to the right. During the examination, an involuntary movement was noted during which his right upper limb flexed whilst the right lower limb extended and his head and eyes deviated to the right. This resolved spontaneously after a couple of minutes.

Investigation showed:

- Hb 9.5g/dL, WCC 3.9×10^9/L, platelets 40×10^9/L.
- CT brain scan with contrast: cerebral oedema.
- LP: CSF opening pressure >40cm H_2O, protein 0.5g/L, glucose 2.5mmol/L (plasma 6mmol/L), 20 WCC/mm^3 (18/mm^3 lymphocytes).

The causative organism (with thanks to Dr Nicola Jones) is shown in Fig. 7.1.

Questions

7a) What is the diagnosis? Describe the characteristic neurological features of this condition and the complications that may occur.

7b) What are the possible brain imaging findings in this condition?

7c) Why has this patient developed this condition?

7d) Which other organ systems may be involved?

7e) What treatment would you give?

7f) Which clinical features influence the prognosis?

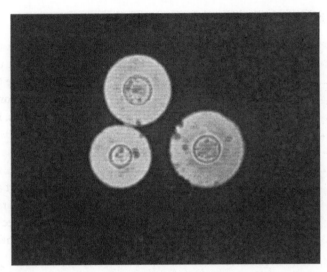

Fig. 7.1

Answers

7a) The organism shown is *Cryptococcus neoformans*, an encapsulated yeast, stained with indian ink.

Cryptococcus neoformans is the third most common CNS infection, after HIV encephalitis and toxoplasma, in patients with advanced HIV infection (CD_4 counts of less than 200/μL), affecting 10% of such patients, and is thus the most common HIV-related CNS fungal infection. It also occurs in patients with other defects in cell-mediated immunity (cf PML, see page 87) e.g. post-transplantation (see page 227), sarcoid and lymphoproliferative disorders). Infection may also occur rarely in subjects without predisposing factors. Laboratory tests including ESR may be normal and eosinophilia is rare.

Neurological complications of *Cryptococcus* infection include:

- Hydrocephalus
- Cranial neuropathy
- Visual loss
- Vasculitis and stroke
- Seizures
- Movement disorders and myoclonus.

Meningitis (usually subacute) is the most common manifestation of cryptococcal CNS infection. Headache, stiff neck and photophobia may occur but are absent in many cases and personality change, cognitive impairment, cranial neuropathy or coma may be the presenting features. Waxing and waning of symptoms with asymptomatic periods may be seen over weeks and months in those with a more chronic course. Cranial neuropathy causing diplopia, decreased visual acuity and facial numbness is seen. Seizures are usually a late feature.

Physical findings are non-specific: patients may be afebrile with minimal or no neck stiffness. Papilloedema occurs in around one third and cranial nerve palsy in about one fifth. Visual loss may occur secondary to fungal infection of the optic tracts, chorioretinitis or raised intracranial pressure. Choreoathetoid movements and myoclonic jerks may be seen but focal motor or sensory symptoms are rare. Dementia may be caused by direct organism involvement of the brain or by hydrocephalus. CSF may be normal in HIV-infected patients as the immune suppression prevents an inflammatory response. Alternatively, there may be elevated protein, depressed glucose and pleocytosis (rarely eosinophilic) with lymphocyte predominance. Indian ink staining for organisms has relatively low sensitivity (25–50% of samples are positive) and thus a negative stain does not rule out infection. Where staining is negative, large volumes of CSF should be sent for culture, which takes 4–6 weeks. Even cultures may sometimes be falsely negative. Serological tests for cryptococcal antigen may be performed on both blood and CSF and have sensitivities of greater than 90% but false negatives and positives do occur. CAF testing for cryptococcal antigen should also be performed.

There are two varieties of *Cryptococcus neoformans*: *Cryptococcus neoformans* var. *neoformans* (and *Cryptococcus neoformans* var. *grubii*) and *Cryptococcus neoformans* var. *gattii*. The latter tends to affect patients without predisposing factors and is prevalent in tropical subtropical countries and rarely affects HIV patients. It more often causes cerebral and pulmonary mass lesions, enhancing lesions on MRI and hydrocephalus. Patients with *C. neoformans* var. *neoformans* are usually immunosuppressed with evidence of diffusely disseminated disease (positive blood and urine cultures) and mortality is higher.

7b) CT or MRI findings in *Cryptococcus* infection include:

- Normal scan
- Cerebral atrophy
- Cerebral oedema
- Mass lesion(s).

Radiological findings in *Cryptococcal* CNS disease are varied and imaging may be normal, or reveal diffuse atrophy (often the only finding in HIV patients), cerebral oedema or mass lesions (usually in immunocompetent patients with the gattii subtype) which may enhance or not. Hypodense lesions on CT, seen as non-enhancing hyperintense lesions on T2–weighted MRI, may be present in the basal ganglia and are thought to correspond to the gelatinous pseudocysts seen on histopathology. These non-enhancing parenchymal cryptococcomas may be associated with non-enhancing, hyperintense dilated perivascular Virchow-Robin spaces. Mass lesions may resemble pyogenic, nocardial, aspergillus, TB, toxoplasma, lymphoma, and other neoplastic lesions. Small enhancing nodules in the parenchyma or subarachnoid are more commonly seen with *Cryptococcus neoformans* var. *gattii*.

7c) This patient was HIV-positive. It was thought that he contracted HIV from the blood transfusion he received abroad since he had no other risk factors for infection. HIV infection probably explains his thrombocytopaenia.

7d) Other organ systems affected by *Cryptococcus* infection are:

- Lungs
- Skin
- Prostate, rarely kidney
- Heart
- Joints
- Eye
- Adrenal glands
- Liver and spleen.

In HIV-positive patients, infection is often disseminated with multiple organ systems being affected but in non-immunosuppressed patients disease tends to be more localized. In general, a careful search for disease in other organ systems should be undertaken as this may be asymptomatic and blood, sputum and urine cultures should always be sent together with cultures from any extraneural lesions. Conversely, a lumbar puncture to look for occult CNS infection should be performed in patients presenting with disease outside the CNS. Pulmonary cryptococcosis may be asymptomatic but cough and dyspnoea may be the presenting features in 5–28% of those with HIV-related cryptococcal infection, and in these patients severe rapidly progressive infection may ensue. In non-immunosuppressed patients, pulmonary cryptococcosis may be stable for long periods or regress spontaneously. Examination findings are often sparse and crackles, pleural rubs and pleural effusions are rare. The CXR may show no obvious abnormality, but in non-AIDS patients, single or multiple circumscribed masses or nodules without hilar involvement, may be seen usually in the upper lobes. Rarely other patterns including segmental pneumonia, and generalized miliary disease are seen. In general, the clinical and radiographic findings are non-specific and cannot be distinguished from *Pneumocystis carinii*, TB, *Histoplasma capsulatum* and various other organisms. Infection may be confirmed by bronchoalveolar lavage and washings or transbronchial biopsy as well as sputum culture.

Single or multiple painless skin lesions are found in 5–10% of patients often affecting the face or scalp. Lesions may appear as papules, pustules, erythematous indurated plaques, soft cutaneous masses or ulcers and may resemble lesions found in numerous other disorders including syphilis, sarcoid, and molluscum contagiosum. Skin biopsy provides rapid diagnosis since organisms are present in large numbers and are easy to identify. Osteolytic bone lesions occur in 5–10%. Skin and bone lesions are seen most commonly in patients with co-existent sarcoid. Prostate involvement occurs more commonly in those with AIDS and the presence of peripheral nodules may resemble tumour. Involvement of other organ systems may occur but is rare.

7e) Treatment length depends on whether or not patients are immunosuppressed.

Immunosuppressed patients, particularly those with HIV, require long term therapy since in the absence of such therapy, relapse rates approach 50%. Initial therapy is usually with combination antifungal treatment given intravenously for 6 weeks. In the current patient with low platelet count, flucytosine was replaced with a larger amphotericin dose owing to its haematological toxicity. This is curative in the majority of non-immunosuppressed patients but relapses may occur and patients should be re-evaluated over the first year. Patients with AIDS require ongoing maintenance with fluconazole or voriconazole. Antiretroviral therapy should be given once the patient is stabilized on antifungal treatment.

CNS masses regress very slowly over months and years (and may even enlarge initially with treatment) but there is no evidence for prolonging therapy in these patients or that surgery is of benefit. There are no randomized trials of steroids in severe acute CNS infection and although temporary improvement might result, long-term therapy interferes with organism clearance from the CNS. There are anecdotal reports that serial LPs, ventriculostomy, acetazolamide and other measures to reduce intracranial pressure are of benefit in patients with visual loss but this has not been confirmed in trials. Hydrocephalus requires shunting.

7f) Prognosis is worse in immunosuppressed patients, older patients, those with disseminated infection, altered conscious level, high titres of cryptococcal antigen in blood or CSF, and low CSF cell counts. Mortality is around 25–30% in acute cryptococcal CNS infection in AIDS. Forty per cent of survivors have residual neurologic deficits including personality change, cranial neuropathy and visual loss. Hydrocephalus may occur as a late complication even after cure and require shunting.

Futher reading

Collazos J (2003). Opportunistic infections of the CNS in patients with AIDS: diagnosis and management. *CNS Drugs*; **17**(12):869–887.

Marra CM (1999). Bacterial and fungal brain infections in AIDS. *Semin Neurol*; **19**(2):177–184.

Mitchell DH, Sorrell TC, Allworth AM (1995). Cryptococcal disease of the CNS in immunocompetent hosts: influence of cryptococcal variety on clinical manifestations and outcome. *Clin Infect Dis*; **20**(3):611–616.

Case 8

A 38-year-old man presented to the emergency department complaining of unsteadiness and dizziness and a fall in which he suffered a minor head injury with no loss of consciousness. No abnormality was found on examination and a skull X-ray was unremarkable. He re-presented 1 week later with a further minor head injury without loss of consciousness and reported ongoing unsteadiness and dizziness, difficulty walking and blurred vision, and was admitted to hospital. He worked as a chemistry laboratory technician and occupied an office containing discarded experimental equipment. Past medical history included investigation for diarrhoea and possible malabsorbtion (for which he had been put on a gluten-free diet). Examination revealed symmetrical incoordination consistent with cerebellar dysfunction and bilateral nystagmus on lateral gaze.

The following investigations were normal:

- CT brain scan,
- FBC, ESR, U&E, TFT, LFT,
- B12, folate,
- CXR, and MRI brain.
- MCV was 100fL.

On examination one week after admission, he was noted to have a strange affect and was talkative but not unwell. He complained of poor memory, blurred vision, fatigue, and inability to concentrate. His hearing was reduced on the right more than the left, the limbs were normal but his coordination was still impaired.

Questions

8a) List 4 possible diagnoses linked to his past medical history of diarrhoea and malabsorbtion that would explain his current symptoms.

8b) What are the clinical features of these 4 conditions?

8c) The actual diagnosis was related to his work as a laboratory technician – what is it?

8d) Which profession was traditionally associated with this disorder?

8e) What tests would you perform to confirm the diagnosis?

Answers

8a) Diagnoses linked to diarrhoea and malabsorbtion causing neurological abnormality include:

- Vitamin E deficiency
- Coeliac disease
- Whipple's disease
- Pellagra (nicotinic acid deficiency)
- Alcohol excess.

This patient had been investigated for malabsorbtion in the past and had been prescribed a gluten-free diet. Several conditions associated with malabsorbtion may cause similar clinical features to those presented in this case. First, **vitamin E deficiency**, usually occurring secondary to chronic fat malabsorbtion, results in neurological abnormalities in both central and peripheral nervous systems. The symptoms and signs mimic those seen in **Friedrich's ataxia**: progressive gait ataxia and limb incoordination, dysarthria, opthalmoplegia, extensor plantars with absent leg reflexes, and marked impairment of vibration and position sense. Variable improvement is seen after vitamin E replacement. **Abetalipoproteinaemia** (Bassen-Kornzweig syndrome) is a rare familial form of malabsorbtion in which there is a neurological syndrome similar to that seen in other vitamin E deficiency states as well as spiky red blood cells (acanthocytes) and retinal pigmentary changes. Isolated vitamin E deficiency without malabsorbtion may be inherited in an autosomal recessive manner.

Coeliac disease has numerous neurological manifestations even in the absence of demonstrable malabsorbtion of nutrients. Age of onset is in the first decade or between 40 and 50-years, and women are affected more than men. As many as 36% of adult patients are reported to have neurological manifestations, most commonly cerebellar ataxia, myoclonus and dementia, and seizures occur in about 5%. Cerebral calcification may be seen on CT brain scan. Neuromuscular manifestations include polymyositis, dermatomyositis (see page 22) and inclusion body myositis with inflammatory features (proximal weakness, high CK and necrosis on muscle biopsy). Sensorimotor axonal neuropathy has been documented. Gluten sensitivity is common and should be looked for in all patients with a relevant unexplained neurological disorder.

Whipple's disease is a chronic multisystem disease that usually affects middle-aged men (80%) with a mean age of onset of 50 years. The causative agent appears to be *Tropheryma whippelii* whose rod shaped structures can be found in mesenteric lymph nodes. The presence of macrophages staining magenta with periodic acid-Schiff (PAS) is the histological hallmark. It is characterized by abdominal pain, steatorrhea and weight loss. Arthritis, fever and lymphadenopathy may also occur. Neurological manifestations are uncommon, occurring in around 5–10% of cases, but may occur in the absence of gastrointestinal symptoms. Dementia (most common), depression, abnormalities of eye movement, other movement disorders including myoclonus and facial muscle twitching, and cerebellar, spinal cord, basal ganglia and hypothalamus involvement, seizures and coma have been recorded. Myopathy and peripheral neuropathy have also been described, which multifocal involvement can therefore resemble a sarcoidosis or vasculitis. Diagnosis requires duodenal biopsy to demonstrate the histolological changes and the typical macrophages and to enable PCR. Treatment is long term with antibiotics that cross the blood–brain barrier eg benzylpenicillin, streptomycin, or cefalosporins. There is a variable response to treatment which needs to be long term and relapse may occur on stopping antibiotics.

Pellagra, a deficiency of nicotinic acid or its precursor tryptophan is uncommon nowadays except in chronic alcoholics and institutionalized patients. It causes nausea, vomiting, diarrhoea and rash, and abnormalities of central and peripheral nervous systems. Irritability, insomnia, depression, confusion, memory impairment, intellectual deterioration, extrapyramidal and cerebellar deficits may develop. The optic and peripheral nerves may be involved. Occasionally there is a myelopathy with extensor plantar responses. The neuronal changes are resistant to niacin treatment suggesting that the full syndrome may be caused by deficiency of several of the B group vitamins. **Chronic alcohol excess** in the absence of pellagra could also cause malabsorbtion secondary to chronic pancreatitis, cerebellar damage and cognitive impairment (see page 18). However, there was nothing to indicate alcohol excess in this patient.

8c) The diagnosis is **mercury poisoning** from inhalation of mercury vapour.

The patient kept a bucket of broken thermometers in his office and played with the mercury from the thermometers during idle moments at work. This would have created a vapour of inorganic mercury in his office. Exposure to inorganic mercury, which is poorly absorbed from the gastrointestinal tract and is absorbed through inhalation, usually occurs during smelting, or after exposure to liquid mercury e.g. in dentists who spill mercury during preparation of dental amalgam. Mercury vapour is also released by dental fillings particularly in those who chew gum but definite adverse affects from this level of exposure are unproven.

Organic mercury intoxication usually results from ingestion of methyl mercury from contaminated fish or grain: epidemics have occurred in Japan (**Minamata disease**) where industrial mercury pollution of sea water resulted in poisoning and deaths in hundreds of people who consumed fish from the contaminated water, and in Iraq after methylmercury coated grain was used to make bread. Another form of organic mercury, ethyl mercury is used as a preservative in vaccines given to infants but there is no proof of adverse effects from the small amount of exposure this entails. Rarely, chemists have been exposed to highly toxic organic mercury compounds such as dimethylmercury which is rapidly absorbed through the skin and by inhalation, with death occurring in all cases.

The symptoms and signs of mercury poisoning are subtly different according to the form in which the mercury was absorbed. **Inorganic mercury** vapour causes a toxic encephalopathy with tremor and bizarre behaviour being the main features. Paraesthaesia, proteinuria and, at high levels, pneumonitis, have also been reported. Methylmercury causes visual field constriction, hearing loss, sensory disturbance, ataxia, tremor, dementia, and psychosis. Ethylmercury causes a similar picture to methylmercury with the addition of acute tubular necrosis. Treatment for inorganic poisoning is with a chelator, meso-2,3-dimercaptosuccinic acid, but this is ineffective in organic poisoning.

Neuropathological studies (mainly in organic mercury poisoning) have shown extensive neuronal death in the cortices especially the calcarine cortex, the cerebellum and the peripheral nervous system with secondary degeneration of directly connected fibre tracts.

8d) Mercury was used in hat making.

Hat makers used inorganic mercury hence the terms 'mad as a hatter' and 'hatter's shakes' and the character of the Mad Hatter in *Alice in Wonderland*.

8e) Blood and urine mercury levels should be requested.

In this patient, blood mercury was 30µg/L (normal range <5µg/L) and urine mercury was 34 µml/L (normal range <5µml/L).

Further reading

Clarkson TW, Magos L, and Myers G-J (2003). The toxicology of mercury - current exposures and clinical manifestations. *NEJM*; **349**(18):1731–1737.

Eto K (2000). Minamata disease. *Neuropathology*; **20** Suppl S14–19. Review.

Nierenberg DW, Nordgren RE, Chang MB, *et al* (1998). Delayed cerebellar disease and death after accidental exposure to dimethylmercury. *NEJM*; **338**:1672–1676.

Case 9

A 30-year-old Polish man was admitted to hospital with confusion and aggressive behaviour. The history was obtained from friends. He had been unwell for the previous 5 days with fever and headache and over the 2 days prior to admission had suffered several episodes of vomiting and complained of a stiff neck. He had been working in the UK as a labourer for the preceding year and had not left the UK during that period. His wife had remained in Poland. None of his friends or workmates had been unwell. He had had one or two brief sexual relationships since his arrival in the UK. There was no past medical history.

On examination, he was uncooperative, agitated and aggressive with confused speech, according to his friends. The temperature was elevated at 37.9°C but general systems examination was otherwise unremarkable. There was neck stiffness and mild photophobia but no focal neurological abnormality.

Investigations showed:

- Hb 15g/dL, WCC 8.2×10^9/L, plt 211×10^9/L
- Na 133mmol/L, K 3.2mm/L, urea 6.0mmol/L and Cr 130μmol/L.
- CRP 22mg/L
- CXR: normal
- CT brain: normal
- LP: CSF opening pressure 32cm H_2O, colourless appearance, WCC 488/mm^3 (64 polymorphs, 424 lymphocytes, 46 red blood cells), protein 2.04g/L, glucose 1.1mmol/L (5.5mmol/L blood), no organisms seen on gram stain, AFB stain negative, Indian ink stain negative.

Initial treatment was with ceftriaxone and aciclovir. The day after admission he was more settled but developed a complete left ptosis with a fixed and dilated pupil and inability to adduct, elevate or abduct the left eye. His condition was otherwise unchanged.

Further investigations showed:

- CT brain with contrast: normal.
- Repeat LP: 770 white cells/mm^3 (70 polymorphs, 700 lymphocytes and 30 red blood cells).

Questions

9a) What is the most likely diagnosis and why?

9b) What might MRI of the brain show?

9c) Which other investigation would you perform and why?

9d) How would you treat this patient?

Answers

9a) The most likely diagnosis is **TB meningitis**.

This previously well man presented with a 5-day history of being unwell with fever and headache followed by encephalopathy manifesting as altered behaviour and cognition. The lumbar puncture opening pressure was raised and there was a CSF pleocytosis with lymphocyte predominance, elevated protein and low glucose. No organisms were seen. This clinical picture could be caused by mycobacteria, listeria, syphilis, brucella, fungal, parasitic or viral infection. Other bacteria associated with CNS infection (e.g. *N. meningitidis*) tend to produce a neutrophilic turbid CSF, although a lymphocyte predominance may be seen in early infection. In pyogenic meningitis, organisms are seen on gram stain in 60–90% of cases provided that antibiotics have not been given prior to lumbar puncture.

The most likely diagnosis, given the clinical features and the CSF findings, is **TB meningitis**. TB causes three different CNS syndromes including meningitis, intracranial tuberculoma (abscess), and spinal arachnoiditis. In TB meningitis, there is typically a prodrome lasting around 2–3 weeks of malaise, fever, headache, fatigue and sometimes altered personality. This is followed by meningism, vomiting, confusion, cranial nerve palsies, occurring in around 20% of cases (the III nerve is the most commonly affected followed by the VI nerve) and long tract signs. There is progression to stupor, coma, and seizures, and death usually occurs within 5–8 weeks of onset in the untreated patient. Atypically, the prodrome may be very long with slowly progressive dementia over months or years, or very short or absent such that the clinical features mimic pyogenic bacterial meningitis. Patients may be categorized into 3 clinical stages: stage I comprises conscious rational patients without focal signs or hydrocephalus; stage II with confusion and/or focal neurological signs; and stage III with coma, delirium, or dense hemiplegia or paraplegia. Stage I has the best, and stage III the worst, prognosis.

Pathologically, organisms in the brain and subarachnoid space induce a hypersensitivity reaction and hence an inflammatory exudate that is always most marked at the base of the brain (basal meningitis) and the optic chiasm. Vasculitis is common with thrombosis and haemorrhagic infarction. Impaired CSF flow and resorption may occur leading to communicating hydrocephalus. Rarely, the hydrocephalus is obstructive when the aqueduct becomes blocked by exudates.

Diagnosis of TB meningitis may be difficult as CSF staining for AFB is often negative (only around 10% of CSF samples are positive for AFB) and cultures may take up to 6 weeks before growth is detectable (cultures were positive after 4 weeks in this patient). TB PCR may be used but false negative and false positive rates are high. Clues include recent exposure to TB, signs of abnormality on general systems examination including lymphadenopathy and splenomegaly and/or on CXR, alcoholism, head injury and immunosuppression. The CSF is not usually turbid and shows an elevated protein, usually 1–5g/L and low glucose (less than half the blood glucose). Very early in infection, there may be a predominance of polymorphs but usually there are 100–500 cells/mm^3 most of which are lymphocytes. Cytological examination shows a subacute meningitic exudate.

Viral infection, particularly with **herpes simplex virus** (see page 6), may produce a similar clinical picture to that seen in the above case, but one would not expect such a high CSF protein or low glucose (the CSF glucose is usually normal or only slightly reduced). Although one would expect to see lymphocyte predominance in the CSF in viral meningoencephalitis, cytologic examination shows a different mixture of cell types to that seen with mycobacteria. Cranial nerve palsies are rare. *Listeria monocytogenes* infection causes a rhomboencephalitis that may present with clinical features similar to those described in this case i.e. headache, fever, vomiting, seizures and focal neurological deficits, including cranial nerve palsies. However, this is a non- meningitic syndrome and there are few or no cells in the CSF and CSF Gram stain and culture are negative. Listeria may also cause a meningitis in which organisms are present on CSF culture. Listeria monocytogenes is a common pathogen in immunosuppressed individuals, pregnant women and neonates, but may also cause infection in the normal host.

The fungus **cryptococcus** (see page 42) could cause a similar clinical picture to that seen in this case and is known to cause cranial neuropathy. The negative indian ink stain on CSF does not exclude infection. Brain imaging is usually abnormal in immunocompetent hosts with CNS cryptococcosis (but may be normal in the immunocompromised patient). Brain imaging is usually abnormal in other fungal infections such as **aspergillus** (see page 295) and **parasitic infection**. There are no clinical features of this case to suggest **Lyme disease** but this should always be considered in patients with a meningoencephalitis, particularly if cranial nerve palsies are present (see page 94). In Lyme disease there may be a CSF pleocytosis but the cell count is usually <200/mm^3, protein <1g/L, and the CSF glucose is rarely depressed.

Cerebral venous sinus thrombosis should be included in the differential diagnosis (see page 10). However, although the CSF pressure was high in this case as one would expect, the CSF protein and number of lymphocytes is higher than is usually the case in this condition although does not completely exclude it. Venous sinus thrombosis may also occur as a complication of CNS infection.

9b) Brain imaging findings in TB meningitis are variable and correlate with disease severity.

CT brain is normal in around 30% of patients with stage I tuberculous meningitis (headache, normal conscious level and no focal neurological signs) but in only 8% of those with stage II disease (focal neurological signs or confusion). It is nearly always abnormal in those with stage III disease (coma). Abnormalities include hydrocephalus and basal enhancement indicating basal exudates (see Fig. 9.1). In general, brain imaging findings are of prognostic significance: complete recovery is the norm in those with normal imaging whereas severe basal exudate is associated with a poor prognosis.

As well as meningitis, TB may cause intracerebral tuberculomas which may present as space occupying lesions or there may be white matter abnormalities (see Figs. 9.1 and 9.2).

9c) HIV testing should be performed.

Co-infection with HIV appears to predispose to extrapulmonary manifestations of TB, and consequently TB meningitis and tuberculoma are seen more commonly in patients with HIV than in those without. HIV is becoming an increasing problem in eastern Europe. The patient described above had also been physically separated from his wife for a prolonged period and had had several other sexual contacts.

9d) Treatment includes:

- Antituberculous antibiotics

- Consideration of steroids.

Early recognition of central nervous system tuberculosis is of paramount importance as the response to therapy depends on the severity of disease at the time of initiation of treatment. Therapy should be started in any patient with a meningitic syndrome and evidence of TB elsewhere in the body, those at high risk of TB, or where prompt evaluation fails to establish an alternative diagnosis. Drug treatment should be on the basis of local patterns of disease and drug resistance: in the UK, combination therapy with isoniazid, rifampicin and pyrazinamide is standard.

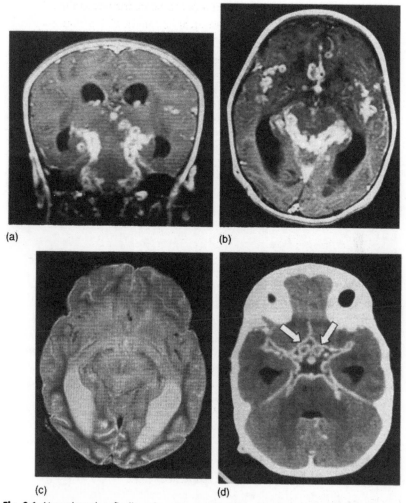

(a)　　　　　　　　　　　　(b)

(c)　　　　　　　　　　　　(d)

Fig. 9.1 Neuroimaging findings in a 2-year-old child with TB: contrast enhanced MRI [coronal and axial (a and b respectively)] showing extensive enhancement of the subarachnoid space consistent with multiple tuberculomas. Axial T2-weighted MRI (c) showing oedema of the cerebral peducles and temporal lobes and CT (d) showing contrast enhancement of the optic nerves (arrows).

If the patient has acquired TB in an area of high resistance, the use of four different drugs (including ethambutol) would be reasonable. There is some evidence to support the use of steroids which may be most beneficial in those with increased intracranial pressure, cerebral oedema, focal neurological deficits, reduced conscious level, and hydrocephalus.

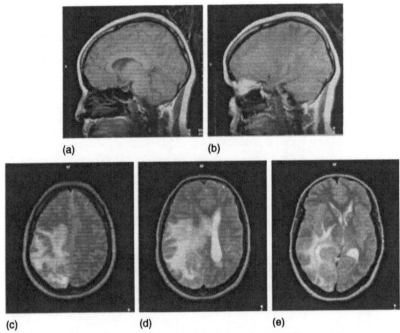

(a) (b)

(c) (d) (e)

Fig. 9.2 Coronal T1 MRI (upper images) showing swelling of the posterior corpus callosum and T2-weighted axial MRI (lower images) showing an extensive oedematous pathology affecting the white matter of the right hemisphere in a Somali man with intracerebral TB. The differential diagnosis for this appearance includes PML (see page 85), glioma, metastasis, and necrotising leukoencephalopathy. A vasculitis might be expected to affect both the white and grey matter.

In practice, steroids are commonly given to patients presenting with stage II or stage III TB meningitis but not to those with stage I disease in whom the prognosis is excellent. Surgical treatment of hydrocephalus may be necessary.

Further reading

Berger JR (1994). Tuberculous meningitis. *Curr Opin Neurol*; 7(3):191–200.

Braun MN, Byers RH, Heyward WL *et al* (1990). Acquired immunodeficiency syndrome and extrapulmonary tuberculosis in the United States. *Arch Intern Med*; **150**:1913

Quagliarello V (2004). Adjunctive steroids for tuberculous meningitis–more evidence, more questions. *N Engl J Med*; **351**(17):1792–1794. No abstract available.

Thwaites GE, Nguyen DB, Nguyen HD *et al* (2004). Dexamethasone for the treatment of tuberculous meningitis in adolescents and adults. *N Engl J Med*; **351**(17):1741–1751.

Case 10

A 70-year-old man developed episodes of rhythmic shaking (approximately 3Hz) of the left arm lasting for up to 2 minutes and preceeded by a brief period of light-headedness. Occasionally, the left arm shaking was accompanied by an odd feeling but no shaking in the left leg. Attacks occurred a few times a week and were almost always triggered by standing up. Consciousness was never impaired. There was a history of hypertension and type II diabetes and he was taking metformin and antihypertensive medication.

On examination there was no abnormality except that he was overweight with an elevated blood pressure of 180/90mm Hg.

Questions

10a) What is the most likely diagnosis, and why?

10b) How would you confirm your diagnosis?

10c) What is the mechanism of such attacks?

10d) What treatments might you suggest?

Answers

10a) The most likely diagnosis is 'limb shaking TIA'

Limb shaking TIA, an uncommon manifestation of focal cerebral ischaemia, is characterized by shaking, jerking or swinging of the limb or limbs on one side of the body or occasionally bilaterally and may be mistaken for focal motor seizures. Dystonic posturing, chorea/athetosis and hemiballismus have also been reported. The jerking or shaking movements do not show a Jacksonian march, tonic contraction or tonic-clonic jerking and secondary generalization does not occur. EEG-recordings during attacks show focal slow waves rather than epileptiform discharges and anticonvulsants are ineffective.

The postural nature of limb shaking TIAs, which are often brought on by sitting or standing up and relieved by lying down, is an important pointer to the aetiology of the attacks, although there may be no measurable postural drop in blood pressure. A more upright posture reduces cerebral blood flow both in normal subjects and in patients with occlusive cerebrovascular disease. Limb shaking TIA is almost always associated with severe carotid disease and thus high stroke risk but has also been reported in Moya Moya disease and aortitis with innominate artery occlusion.

There is little in this patient's history to support a diagnosis of **focal motor seizures** and the relationship of the shaking episodes to posture and the lack of secondary generalization make seizures unlikely. **Hypoglycaemia** should be considered in any diabetic patient with possible seizures but it does not occur with metformin.

10b) Confirmation of the diagnosis of limb shaking TIA requires demonstration of a vascular lesion affecting blood supply to the relevant cerebral hemisphere and exclusion of seizure activity.

Most commonly an occlusive lesion of the carotid is seen in association with limb shaking TIA but other vascular lesions may be present such as those caused by Moya Moya disease (multifocal intracerebral vascular occlusion with collateral formation) or tumour invasion of a vessel such as the carotid artery.

In this patient, CT brain and EEG were normal but carotid duplex showed an occluded right internal carotid artery and 60% stenosis of the left internal carotid artery. Reduced flow in the right middle cerebral artery (18cm/sec vs. 55cm/sec for right and left respectively) was confirmed on transcranial Doppler ultrasonography.

10c) Current evidence suggests that a focal haemodynamic abnormality is likely to be responsible for the development of limb shaking TIA.

Limb shaking TIAs often improve after revascularization procedures or reduction in antihypertensive therapy. Cerebral blood flow and vasomotor reactivity (indicating reserve dilatory capacity of cerebral resistance vessels) are reduced to a greater extent in patients with as compared to those without limb shaking TIA. Spontaneous improvement of vasomotor reactivity and also of symptoms may occur presumably as a result of collateral growth since reduced cerebral vasoreactivity is associated with a poor collateral network.

Severe occlusive disease of the internal carotid artery/ies primarily causes reduction in perfusion of the ipsilateral limb motor cortical areas (middle cerebral artery/anterior cerebral artery watershed), hence the lack of reports of facial twitching in association with limb shaking TIA. Similar but smaller changes occur in the contralateral borderzone owing to diversion of blood via the anterior communicating artery. This would account for the bilateral limb shaking observed in some patients. Interestingly, interruption of speech and verbal paraphrasic errors have been reported in association with limb shaking attacks. This may represent hypoperfusion of Wernicke's area which lies close to the anterior/posterior circulation watershed.

10d) Management of limb shaking TIA focuses on maintaining or improving cerebral blood flow and reducing the risk of stroke.

Reducing antihypertensive therapy will increase cerebral blood flow and improve symptoms but is not ideal in vascular patients. More aggressive anti-hypertensive therapy is possible after surgical revascularization procedures which are also effective in improving or abolishing symptoms. Carotid stenosis should be treated by endarterectomy. In the case of carotid occlusion, extracranial–intracranial bypass surgery may be performed for relief of symptoms but there is no evidence that it reduces the risk of stroke.

Further reading

Baumgartner RW, Baumgartner I (1998). Vasomotor reactivity is exhausted in transient ischaemic attacks with limb shaking. *J Neurol Neurosurg Psychiatry*; 65(4):561–564.

Khan A, Beletsky V, Kelley R, *et al.* (1999). Orthostatic-mediated hypoperfusion in limb-shaking transient ischemic attack. *J Neuroimaging*; 9(1):43–44.

Zaidat OO, Werz MA, Landis DM, *et al.* (1999). Orthostatic limb shaking from carotid hypoperfusion. *Neurology*; 53(3):650–651

Case 11

A 50-year-old female factory worker was referred to the admitting medical team by the duty police surgeon. The police had been called to her house during the night by her husband after she had begun acting in a violent and agitated manner. She was convinced that there were intruders in the house and had chased her husband round the house with a knife thinking that he was one of them. On arrival on the medical admissions unit in the afternoon of the following day, she was behaving normally and was able to answer questions although she had poor recollection of the events overnight. She remained convinced that there had been intruders in her house, but was aware that she might have been hallucinating at times. She described being unwell for the preceding 4 days with vomiting and abdominal pain that was central and constant but this had largely resolved. She had also been constipated.

She had had one previous admission 6 months previously for vomiting and abdominal pain. Endoscopic examination was normal. There was a past history of hypertension, gout, osteoarthritis of the left hip, and increased alcohol intake. There was no known family history. She was taking atenolol, tramadol, lansoprazole, and aspirin, and denied illegal drug use.

On examination, she was apyrexial, pulse 90/min and BP 100/63 mmHg. There was no abdominal abnormality, neck stiffness, or photophobia. MTS was 9/10 with no focal neurological abnormality. There was some scarring over the knuckles of both hands and the suggestion of early blister formation.

Investigations showed:

- Hb 12.6g/dL, WCC × 10^9/L, plt139 × 10^9/L
- ESR 11mm/h, CRP<8mg/L
- Na 139mmol/L, K 3.3mmol/L, glc 6.4 g/dL, Cr 152μmol/L
- LFTs normal, amylase 75mmol/L
- ABG on air: pH 7.44, pCO_2 4.23kPa, pO_2 9.64kPa, lactate 3.5 mmol/L, bicarbonate 23.2mmol/L
- Urinalysis: normal
- Abdominal ultrasound: no abnormality seen.

Over the next 2 days, she remained well with no further episodes of disturbed behaviour.

Questions

11a) What is the diagnosis? Which other forms of this condition are associated with neurological abnormalities?

11b) What other neurological abnormalities may occur?

11c) In female sufferers, when might symptoms be more likely to occur?

11d) What further investigations would you request?

11e) What treatment would you advise?

11f) What are the problems with drug treatment of one of the neurological complications of this condition?

Answers

11a) The diagnosis is variegate **porphyria** (caused by a deficiency of protoporphyrin oxidase) or hereditary coproporphyria (caused by coproporhyrin oxidase deficiency). The other acute porphyria, acute intermittent porphyria (see below), causes neurological abnormalities but not skin abnormalities.

The porphyrias are a group of inherited disorders caused by deficiencies of individual enzymes involved in the biochemical pathway of haem synthesis resulting in neuropsychiatric signs, cutaneous signs, or both. They are rare but important because they mimic a number of other diseases and thus may be difficult to diagnose. The porphyrias are classified into acute (hepatic) and non-acute porphyrias.

Acute porphyrias
- Acute intermittent porphyria
- Variegate porphyria
- Hereditary coproporphyria

Non-acute porphyrias
- Porphyria cutanea tarda
- Erythropoietic porphyria
- Congential porphyria

The acute porphyrias present with severe attacks of neurovisceral dysfunction associated with the over production and increased urinary excretion of the porphyrin precursors δ-aminolaevulionic acid (ALA) and porphobilinogen. Patients with variegate and hereditary coproporphyria may also have cutaneous photosensitivity with blistering and scarring of sun exposed areas caused by overproduction of porphyrin. In the non-acute porphyrias, there is overproduction of porphyrins only rather than the precursors and patients have cutaneous manifestations but none of the neurological symptoms. Excess porphyrins are mainly excreted in the faeces via the bile.

   The features of an attack of acute porphyria can all be explained by dysfunction of the autonomic, peripheral and central nervous systems and include gastrointestinal symptoms and neuropsychiatric abnormalities (see below). In the current patient, these features were accompanied by evidence of cutaneous damage on the hands suggesting variegate porphyria or hereditary coproporphyria, rather than acute intermittent porphyria. Of the gastrointestinal manifestations, abdominal pain is the most common and may be severe enough to prompt laparotomy, which may be fatal. The diagnosis of acute porphyria must thus be considered in any patient with unexplained abdominal pain. The pain is usually diffuse and can radiate around to the back. Abdominal examination may be normal or there be mild tenderness diffusely. The abdominal pain is often accompanied by nausea, vomiting and constipation, although rarely diarrhoea may occur. The gastrointestinal symptoms often precede the neuropsychiatric manifestations.

Diagnosis may be suggested by a family history as inheritance is usually autosomal dominant although it may be absent in as much as one third of patients since the condition may remain latent. There is a female preponderance probably owing to hormonal fluctuations precipitating attacks.

11b) The neurological manifestations in acute porphyria include:

- Acute neuropathy
- Neuropsychiatric abnormalities
- Autonomic dysfunction.

The neuropathy may be the presenting feature of an attack and complicates more than 50% of attacks. The predominantly motor involvement is characterised by subacute generalized, proximal or asymmetrical muscle weakness. The arms may be affected before the legs and cranial nerve involvement is common. Sensory impairment may occur either in a distal glove stocking pattern or affecting the upper limbs and trunk (so-called bathing costume distribution). Rarely mononeuritis may be seen.

Symptoms may be rapidly progressive mimicking Guillain–Barré syndrome (see page 76) although the pathology is axonal rather than demyelinating as in the latter, and patients may require respiratory support. There is muscle wasting and tendon jerks are reduced or absent although may be paradoxically retained at the ankles. Weakness may take months to resolve and resolution may be incomplete after a severe attack.

The neuropsychiatric manifestations are common and include psychosis, delusions, mania, hallucinations, and depression. Abnormalities may persist between attacks particularly in children. Seizures may be seen in around 5–20% and may be the presenting feature.

Autonomic dysfunction is evidenced by tachycardia, hypertension, sweating, pyrexia and pallor (and the gastrointestinal symptoms). Urinary retention and hypotension may occur. SIADH may occur causing hyponatraemia and may contribute to the aetiology of seizures and altered mental state.

11c) The hormonal changes of the menstrual cycle mean that some women have a tendency for attacks to occur in the premenstrual phase of the cycle or occasionally at ovulation. Similarly, attacks may be precipitated by pregnancy and the use of oral contraceptives.

11d) The biochemical hallmark of an attack of acute porphyria is the elevation of ALA and porphobilinogen in the urine.

Porphobilinogen causes darkening of the urine, which becomes more apparent when the urine is left to stand and can be used as a bedside test before formal measurement of porphyrin precursors in the urine. Levels of ALA and porphobilinogen may decrease rapidly after an attack in variegate and hereditary coproporphyria but remain elevated in acute intermittent porphyria. In this patient, ALA and porphobilinogen were normal 2 days after the attack. It should be noted that porphyrin metabolism is affected by other factors including lead poisoning, alcohol, liver disease, and certain drugs that may cause elevation of urinary porphyrin precursors. There is faecal excretion of coproporhyrin and of coproporhyrin and protoporphyrin in hereditary coprophophyria and in variegate porphyria respectively, but not in acute intermittent porphyria. The CSF is normal or shows protein elevation. EMG studies are consistent with a predominantly axonal motor neuropathy.

11d) Initial management of the acute attack should be followed by advice to the patient on the avoidance of future attacks and screening of other family members.

Management of the acute attack is generally supportive and includes removal of offending drugs and treatment of intercurrent infection together with the administration of a carbohydrate load. Persistence of neurological deficit for 24 hours after initial management has been started is an indication for treatment with haematin, which suppresses the activity of δ-ALA synthetase.

Attacks may be precipitated by a number of factors including starvation, infection, alcohol and many drugs, including barbiturates, anticonvulsants, and female hormones. Preventive treatment thus includes avoidance of low calorie diets, alcohol, and drugs known to precipitate attacks.

Screening of urine for porphobilinogen will pick up less than 50% of cases of latent acute porphyria and more complex biochemical tests may be required. Screening using molecular biological techniques is difficult, although the chromosomal locations of the enzymatic defects in all the porphyrias is known, as there is marked genetic heterogeneity i.e. multiple different genetic abnormalities occur and amino acid substitutions, splicing defects and premature insertion of stop codons are all seen.

11e) Management of patients with seizures secondary to porphyria or with epilepsy and porphyria is difficult as many of the commonly used drugs, such as phenytoin and sodium valproate, precipitate attacks.

Benzodiazepines and magnesium sulphate are thought to be safe for initial seizure control. Gabapentin has been recommended for seizure prophylaxis as it does not undergo significant hepatic metabolism.

Further reading

Albers KW and Fink JK (2004). Porphyric neuropathy. *Muscle Nerve*; 30(4):410–422. Review.

Elder GH, Hift RJ, Meissner PN (1997). The acute porphyrias. *Lancet*; 349:1613–1617.

Peters TJ and Mills KR (2006). Porphyria for the neurologist: the bare essentials. *Practical Neurology*; 6:255–258.

Peters TJ, Sarkany R (2005). Porphyria for the general physician. *Clinical Med*; 5:275–281.

Scarlett YV and Brenner DA (1998). Porphyrias. *Journal of Clinical Gastroenterology*; 27:192–196.

Case 12

A 54-year-old male sales manager was admitted to hospital for investigation of sudden onset left leg weakness and pins and needles in the left leg and hand lasting for 1 to 2 minutes and occurring up to 4 times a day. He had been investigated 3 years previously following an episode of dysarthria and confusion, at which time an MRI brain scan was reportedly normal and a diagnosis of migraine had been made. There was no other past medical history. His mother had a history of dementia and recurrent strokes in her late sixties and his father had angina. Two sisters were well. He did not smoke and was on no medication.

On examination, he appeared well and general systems were unremarkable. Blood pressure was 130/80 mmHg. He was alert and orientated and examination of the cranial nerves was normal. There was mild left pronator drift, but power was normal in all limbs. Limb reflexes were brisk, particularly on the left, and there was mild left-sided incoordination and bilateral extensor plantars.

Investigations showed:

- Cholesterol 4.5mmol/L, glucose 4.6mm/L
- ECG, carotid ultrasound: normal
- Echocardiogram: mild left ventricular hypertrophy
- T2-weighted MRI brain scan is shown in Fig. 12.1
- CSF examination and visual evoked potentials: normal.

Questions

12a) Describe the MRI abnormalities.

12b) Give a differential diagnosis.

12c) What is the most likely diagnosis and why?

12d) What investigations would you perform in order to confirm the diagnosis?

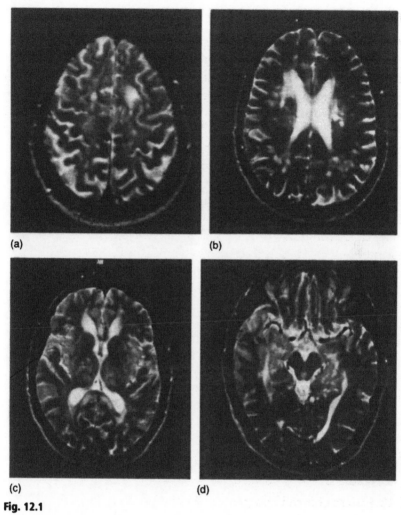

(a)

(b)

(c)

(d)

Fig. 12.1

Answers

12a) The MRI shows focal, diffuse and confluent areas of hyperintensity in the periventricular and subcortical white matter and brainstem (see Fig. 12.2).

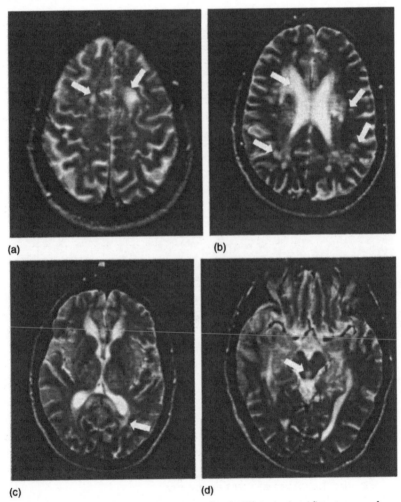

(a)

(b)

(c)

(d)

Fig. 12.2 The axial T2-weighted MRI shows focal, diffuse and confluent areas of hyperintensity (arrows) in the periventricular and subcortical white matter (a,b,c) and brainstem (d).

12b) The differential diagnosis includes:

- CADASIL (cerebral autosomal dominant arteriopathy with subcortical infarcts and leukoencephalopathy)
- Multiple sclerosis (MS)
- Vasculitis.

The history of sudden onset left limb weakness associated with sensory symptoms suggests a cerebrovascular event. The previous episode of sudden onset dysarthria would be consistent with a previous vascular event, possibly in a different arterial territory.

The multifocal white matter lesions seen on MRI could be caused by vascular disease or demyelination. **Sporadic small vessel disease** (narrowing and occlusion of the small perforating vessels of the brain) is a possible diagnosis, although the confusion during the first episode would be unexpected in a patient this age unless there was a thalamic infarct causing memory loss. The absence of vascular risk factors makes sporadic small vessel disease unlikely at this age, although the echocardiogram did show left ventricular hypertrophy indicating possible undiagnosed hypertension (not excluded by a single normal blood pressure measurement). **CADASIL** is discussed below.

Multiple white matter abnormalities, characteristically flame shaped in the periventricular region, round or oval elsewhere, are seen in **multiple sclerosis (MS)** in which sudden onset neurological symptoms may occur. There is often a history of typical MS episodes such as optic neuritis or transverse myelitis. The normal CSF and visual evoked potentials do not exclude MS but they do make this diagnosis less likely. **Cerebral vasculitis** (see page 174) (primary or secondary to systemic vasculitis) may cause multiple CNS lesions and present with stroke-like episodes. However, the patient appeared generally well (small vessel vasculitis often causes an encephalopathy) and MRI abnormalities were restricted to the subcortical areas. **Mitochondrial encephalopathy with stroke-like episodes (MELAS)** (see page 103) causes stroke-like episodes and may be associated with migraine but the MRI abnormalities are usually cortical (often occipital) rather than subcortical and there were no other features to suggest this disorder.

12c) The most likely diagnosis is **CADASIL**.

CADASIL is the most likely diagnosis because of the family history of stroke and dementia, the previous history of a stroke-like episode, associated migraine and subcortical white matter abnormalities on MRI. CADASIL is a rare hereditary (autosomal dominant) condition characterized by migraine with aura, recurrent stroke and TIA (usually lacunar in type), and progressive subcortical dementia. There are usually no vascular risk factors. The occurrence of new mutations has been described, but the vast majority of cases do have a family history.

The first clinical manifestation is often migraine with aura in the third or fourth decade although migraine is not seen in all pedigrees or all members of an affected family. There is a high frequency of basilar and hemiplegic migraine and some patients may have migraine coma (see page 203). Stroke is the most common clinical manifestation, affecting around 85% of subjects and occurring at a mean age of around 50 years. Most of the strokes are lacunar resulting in classical syndromes such as pure motor stroke or ataxic hemiparesis but dysphasia and dysarthria, isolated ataxia, and hemianopia, may be seen.

Dementia is the second most common manifestation of CADASIL, occurring in one-third of patients and at a mean age of 60 years. Frontal features (apathy and loss of executive function) and memory impairment are seen with aphasia and apraxia occurring late. Dementia is always associated with pyramidal signs, pseudobulbar palsy, gait difficulties, and/or urinary incontinence. Mood disturbance affects 20–30% and is usually depression, although bipolar disorder has been observed. Rarely, deafness and seizures may occur (cf. MELAS).

Imaging is always abnormal in symptomatic subjects and shows characteristic focal punctate or nodular hypointensities on T1-weighted MRI and hyperintensities on T2-weighted MRI in the basal ganglia, periventricular and subcortical white matter and sometimes in the brainstem, usually the pons. Cortical and cerebellar lesions are exceptional. White matter changes may be widespread and confluent in advanced cases and severity increases with age.

12d) The diagnosis may be made by:

- Histological examination of skin, muscle or nerve
- Demonstration of a mutation in the *Notch 3* gene.

In CADASIL, the small vessels are affected by a non-arteriosclerotic non-amyloid arteriopathy causing vessel lumen narrowing which is seen in the leptomeningeal and perforating arteries of the brain and also in skin, muscle, liver, kidneys, and spleen. The diagnosis can be made by histological examination of biopsy samples from skin, muscle (Fig. 12.3) or nerve, in which the smooth muscle basal lamina of the small blood vessels is thickened by a granular deposit which appears dense on electron microscopy.

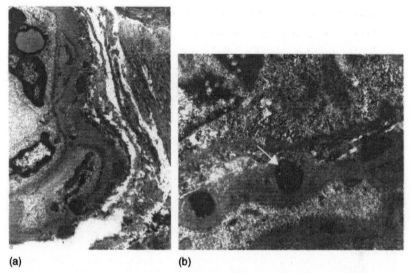

(a)   (b)

Fig.12.3 Electron microscopy of muscle from the patient described in this case showing thickening of the basal lamina of the small blood vessels and presence of dense eosinophilic material (arrow).

The gene causing CADASIL has been identified (*Notch 3*) and mapped to chromosome 19q12. It encodes a transmembrane receptor. Multiple mutations have been reported but most are clustered within two exons and 70% of mutations are detectable by a genetic test currently used in diagnosis.

Further reading

Charbriat H and Bousser MG (2003). CADASIL. Cerebral autosomal dominant arteriopathy with subcortical infarcts and leuloencephalopathy. *Adv Neurol*; **92**:142–150.

Chabriat H, Vahedi K, Iba-Zizen MT, *et al* (1995). Clinical spectrum of CADASIL: a study of 7 families. Cerebral autosomal dominant arteriopathy with subcortical infarcts and leuloencephalopathy. *Lancet*; **346**(8980):934–939.

Dichigans M, Mayer M, Uttner I, *et al* (1998) The phenotypic spectrum of CADASIL: clinical findings in 102 cases. *Annals of Neurology*; **44**(5):731–739.

Joutel A, Vahedi K, Corpechot C, *et al* (1997). Strong clustering and stereotyped nature Notch 3 mutations in CADASIL patients. *Lancet*; **350**:1511–1515.

Case 13

A 34-year-old male vet presented with a 5-day history of fatigue, jaundice, decreased appetite, nausea, and inguinal lymphadenopathy. Three days before admission, he noticed that his urine looked dark and his left foot and the tips of his fingers felt numb and were tingling. The day before admission, he developed a left facial droop and inability to close the left eye. By the day of admission, the numbness and tingling had spread upwards to involve the limbs as far as the knees and elbows, he felt short of breath when talking, was unable to stand, and had choked on some paracetamol. He complained of aching in his lower back. He had had no contacts with jaundiced people, had not been abroad, had not received any blood transfusions in the past, and was married. There was no past medical history and he was a non-smoker and moderate drinker. He was on no medication.

On examination, he was icteric, apyrexial, with a pulse of 70/min regular and BP of 140/70mmHg. There was hepatosplenomegaly and bilateral inguinal lymphadenopathy. Rectal examination was normal. Neurological examination revealed left facial numbness, bilateral VII nerve lower motor neuron palsy and reduced palatal movement. There was generalized muscle weakness, reduced tone and absent reflexes in all limbs. Upper limb sensation was objectively normal but there was reduced pinprick, temperature sensation and joint position sense below the knees. Plantar reflexes were downgoing.

Investigations showed:

- Hb 9.7g/dL, MCV 85 fL, WCC 10.9×10^9/L, plt 205×10^9/L, reticulocyte count 5.8%
- CRP 48mg/L
- Bili 73μmol/L, alb 43g/L, AST 40IU/L, GGT 13IU/L, alk phos 80IU/L, LDH 338IU/L
- U&E, TSH, B12, folate normal
- U/S abdomen: hepatosplenomegaly
- CSF: no cells, protein 0.31g/L, glc 3.4mmol/L (blood 6.5mmol/L).

Questions

13a) What is the neurological diagnosis? Describe the clinical features and modes of presentation of this condition.

13b) Describe the variants of this condition.

13c) Which other conditions may mimic the diagnosis in 13a)?

13d) What haematological problem do the laboratory results suggest?

13e) What is the most likely underlying non neurological condition?

13f) What further bedside test needs to be done urgently in this patient?

13g) What other investigations would you request?

13f) How would you manage this patient?

Answers

13a) The diagnosis is **Guillain–Barré syndrome (GBS).**

GBS is an acute inflammatory demyelinating polyradiculoneuropathy. Inflammatory demyelinating polyradiculoneuropathies (IDPs) can be classified into acute (AIDP or GBS) and chronic forms (CIDP) by their clinical course. In GBS, deficits are maximal over days followed by a plateau phase and eventual recovery, whereas the chronic forms of IDP pursue a slowly progressive or a relapsing and remitting course.

GBS affects all age groups and incidence rates increase with age from 0.8/100000 at 18 years to 3.2/100000 in the over 60s. Approximately two-thirds of patients report a preceding event, most commonly an upper respiratory or gastrointestinal infection, surgery or vaccination 1–4 weeks before the onset of the neurological symptoms although the agent responsible for the prodromal illness is frequently unidentified. Specific infections linked to GBS include *Campylobacter jejuni*, CMV, HIV (see page 263), *Mycoplasma pneumoniae* and EBV, VZV, hepatitis A and B. Associated vaccines include tetanus, diptheria and polio.

Patients commonly present with paraesthesias alone, paraesthesias with weakness or weakness alone. The limb weakness usually begins distally and ascends proximally over hours to days to involve the orofacial, swallowing, and respiratory muscles. Less commonly, the weakness may begin more proximally. Areflexia or hyporeflexia is invariable. Progression should be complete by about 4 weeks; if symptoms continue beyond this point, the condition is subacute IDP or CIDP if relapse and remission occur. Cranial nerve palsies are common and bilateral facial nerve palsies occur in at least 50% of cases (see page 92). Ventilation is required in a significant minority of patients (see below). Sensory signs are usually minor with distal loss of vibration being most common. Pain occurs in the majority and is sometimes severe, usually affecting the thorax, but tingling or burning of the extremities is also seen. Autonomic dysfunction is common in patients admitted to hospital and is manifested by persistent tachycardia, arrhythmia, heart block and rarely asystole, labile hypertension, postural hypotension, urinary retention, and intestinal ileus. Mortality is 5–10% with modern critical care compared to around one third previously.

Routine laboratory investigations are usually unremarkable although mild transaminase elevation may be seen. Rarely glomerulonephritis from immune complex deposition may cause haematuria and proteinuria. ECG changes include ST depression, QT prolongation and QRS widening.

The CSF typically is acellular with increased protein, although the latter may be normal in the week after presentation and occasionally may never become elevated. Extreme elevation of protein may lead to intracranial hypertension and papilloedema. CSF pleocytosis is a characteristic feature of GBS associated with HIV infection (see page 264). NCS show evidence of proximal demyelination sometimes with secondary axonal degeneration. Antiganglioside antibodies (to myelin glycolipids) may be found possibly more commonly with campylobacter infection.

The pathology of GBS is thought to be autoimmune mediated by T cells and antibodies directed at antigens on peripheral nerves. It is thought that preceding infection generates an antibody response to the infecting organism that shares epitopes with the host's peripheral nerves.

13b) There are several variants of GBS:

- Miller Fisher syndrome
- Acute pandysautonomia
- Acute motor axonal neuropathy (AMAN)
- Acute motor sensory axonal neuropathy (AMSAN).

Miller Fisher syndrome is characterized by opthalmoplegia, ataxia and areflexia. Cranial nerves other than the ocular motor nerves may be affected. Anti-ganglioside GQ1b antibodies are found acutely in most patients (and in patients with GBS and opthalmoplegia). Acute pandysautonomia is characterized by combined sympathetic and parasympathetic failure and areflexia without somatic sensory or motor involvement. There are two other variants of GBS in which the neuropathy is axonal rather than demyelinating and which are associated particularly with camplobacter infection, one affecting motor nerves only (acute motor axonal neuropathy (AMAN)) and occurring in epidemics in northern China in the summer, and the other rare form affecting both motor and sensory nerves (acute motor sensory axonal neuropathy (AMSAN)).

13c) There are several other conditions leading to subacute motor weakness that may be difficult to distinguish from GBS (see list below) including acute spinal cord lesions with flaccid paraparesis.

- *Acute neuropathies:*
  - Acute porphyria (see page 65)
  - Diptheria (cranial and peripheral neuropathy occurs some weeks after initial infection)

- Toxins eg lead, neurotoxic fish, shellfish
- Vasculitis
- Inflammatory meningoradiculopathies e.g. Lyme disease (see page 92), CMV.
- *Neuromuscular junction abnormalities:*
  - Botulism, myasthenia gravis.
- *Myopathies:*
  - Rhabdomyolysis (see page 111)
  - Intensive care myopathy
  - Myositis (see page 22)
  - Hypokalaemia, hypophosphataemia.
- *Central nervous system disorders:*
  - Poliomyelitis, rabies
  - Transverse myelitis
  - Acute spinal cord lesion.

13d) The laboratory results show an anaemia with normal MCV, elevated bilirubin and LDH and increased reticulocyte count. This is consistent with haemolysis.

13e) The underlying diagnosis is **EBV infection.**

The diagnosis of GBS should prompt a search for a precipitating condition. As discussed above, EBV is associated with GBS. EBV classically causes fever, anorexia, headache, malaise, and sore throat. Lymphadenopathy (most marked in the cervical region) and splenomegaly are common. Hepatomegaly occurs in 10% and jaundice in 8%. More rarely, myocarditis, encephalitis, meningitis, splenic rupture and autoimmune haemolytic anaemia or thrombocytopaenia may occur.

   CMV and **toxoplasma** may produce a similar clinical picture to EBV but in the former marked lymphadenopathy is rare, and the latter is not known to be associated with GBS. **Primary HIV infection** (see page 263) produces an EBV-like syndrome although rash occurs in 50% unlike in EBV, lymphadenopathy is generalized, and jaundice and haemolysis would be unusual. **Hepatitis A and B** are associated with GBS and cause jaundice, haemolysis but one would expect abnormal liver function tests.

13f) Vital capacity, airway and swallowing function should be monitored.

Vital capacity should be measured regularly in all patients with suspected GBS. In this patient it was 2L (predicted 5.04L) on admission and fell further such that he required ventilation and eventually tracheostomy. Assisted ventilation is required in 12–23% of patients with GBS, and is more commonly required in older patients. Impairment of airway protection is also an indication for intubation.

13g) Further investigations include:

- Haptoglobin, Coombs' test, urinary urobilinogen
- Blood film
- EBV monospot test and IgG and IgM measurement, serology for other antecedent infection as per list above
- Arterial blood gas
- NCS.

In this patient the haptoglobins were reduced at 0.4 g/L (0.5–2.65 g/L), Coombs' test was negative and a bone marrow showed a reactive marrow with no malignant cells. This was felt to support the diagnosis of haemolysis despite the negative Coombs' test. EBV IgM and IgG were positive consistent with recent infection. The monospot test was negative but this is not uncommon in older adults with EBV. NCS showed absent and delayed f waves consistent with GBS.

13h) Treatment is supportive including intensive care for respiratory and cardiovascular support and management of bulbar and airway function.

Tracheal suction may trigger episodes of hypotension, bradycardia or even asystole, owing to autonomic instability. Specific interventions aim to reduce the level of circulating antibody with IVIG or plasma exchange, which have been shown to speed recovery. Steroids have not been shown to be beneficial. Overall, approximately 1.5% of patients with GBS die and more than 10% are dependent at 1 year. The axonal variant of GBS tends to have a worse outcome. Recurrence is rare.

Further reading

Hartung HP, Kieseier BC, Kiefer R (2001). Progress in Guillain–Barré syndrome. *Curr Opin Neurol*; 14(5):597–604.

Hartung HP, Willison HJ, Kieseier BC (2002). Acute immunoinflammatory neuropathy: update on Guillain–Barré syndrome. *Curr Opin Neurol*; 15(5):571–577.

Kieseier BC, Hartung HP (2003). Therapeutic strategies in the Guillain–Barré syndrome. *Semin Neurol*; 23(2):159–168.

Levin KH (2004). Variants and mimics of Guillain–Barré Syndrome. *Neurologist*; 10(2):61–74.

Pritchard J (2006). What's new in Guillain–Barré syndrome? *Pract Neurol*; 6:208–217.

Case 14

A 32-year-old woman was admitted with a 1-week history of fever, headache, speech difficulty, and increasing confusion. There was no past medical or family history of note. She lived with her husband, worked as a shop assistant, was an ex-smoker and did not drink alcohol. She was on no regular medication.

On examination, she was pyrexial at 38°C with a pulse of 120/min, blood pressure 105/60mmHg and a soft systolic murmur at the left sternal edge. There was a facial rash in a butterfly distribution across both cheeks and oral candida. There was no lymphadenopathy. The chest was clear and oxygen saturations were 97% on air. The abdomen was unremarkable. There was a fluctuating drowsiness with a mild expressive dysphasia (unable to name the hands or winder on a watch) and mild confusion (MTS 8/10) with apparent mental slowing. Neck stiffness was absent. Examination of the cranial nerves and limbs was unremarkable.

Investigations showed:

- Hb 11.2g/dL, MCV 84fL, WCC 3.74×10^9/L (polymorphs 2.3×10^9/L, lymphocytes 0.94×10^9/L), platelets 103×10^9/L
- Na 140mmol/L, K 4.3mmol/L, Cr 56μmol/L, glucose 5.3mmol/L, bili 14μmol/L, alb 36g/L, AST 94IU/L, alk phos 49IU/L
- ESR 50mm/h, CRP 7mg/L.

CT brain is shown in Fig. 14.1.

CSF: opening pressure 32cm H_2O, glucose 3g/dL, protein 0.42g/L, RBC 27/mm^3, WCC 1/mm^3, no organisms, no growth.

Urine dipstick: 1+ blood, nil else.

Questions

14a) What does the CT scan show?

14b) Give a differential diagnosis

An MRI scan was performed and is shown in Fig. 14.2 [T2-weighted axial images (a–d) and T1-weighted coronal slice (e) together with the MRA (f)].

14c) What does the MRI scan show?

14d) Give a revised differential diagnosis based on the MRI result. What is the most likely diagnosis?

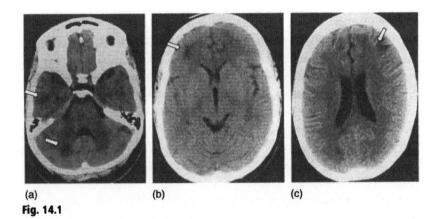

(a)   (b)   (c)

Fig. 14.1

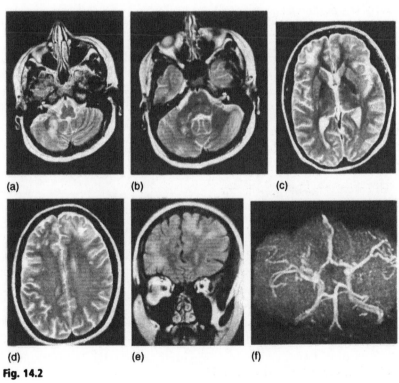

(a)   (b)   (c)

(d)   (e)   (f)

Fig. 14.2

Answers

14a) The CT scan shows low densities particularly deep in the right cerebellum and temporal lobe (see arrows in Fig. 14.1a) and the subcortical frontal regions (see arrows in Figs. 14.1b and 14.1c). The ventricles are not enlarged and there is no evidence of cortical atrophy. These findings are non-specific but could represent areas of infarction, a diffuse encephalitic process or a white matter disease.

14b) The differential diagnosis includes:

- Infection:
  - Viral e.g. herpes simplex virus, VZV, HIV, PML
  - Lyme disease, rickettsia
  - Toxoplasma.
- Multiple strokes
  - Infective endocarditis
  - Vasculitis   —primary e.g. Churg–Strauss
                    —secondary e.g. SLE, sarcoid, TB
  - SLE related cardioembolism or thrombotic tendency
- Acute disseminated encephalomyelitis (ADEM).
- Inherited disorders:
  - MELAS.
- Other:
  - Hashimoto's encephalitis.

The clinical features of fever, headache, drowsiness, confusion and aphasia put CNS infection high on the list of differential diagnoses. The CT findings are non-specific and certainly could not be used to rule out infection such as **herpes simplex type 1** which typically presents with this clinical picture (see page 4). Further, CNS infection may itself cause vasculitis leading to infarction (see below). The LP revealed an elevated opening pressure but the CSF was normal. This does not rule out viral or opportunistic CNS infection but makes pyogenic bacterial or tuberculous infection extremely unlikely. The presence of oral candida could be related to her recent course of antibiotics but would be unusual in a otherwise fit young person. An alternative explanation would be that this patient has an underlying immune deficiency and increases the likelihood of an opportunistic infection.

There are a number of features of this case, that are consistent with **HIV seroconversion**, which typically causes an EBV-like illness 2–6 weeks after virus entry (see page 263). Fever, rash, headache and confusion with mild transaminitis are common (as is lymphadenopathy which was not present in this patient). A number of neurological syndromes may occur, most commonly aseptic meningitis and neuropathy (VII nerve and radiculopathy), but acute demyelination may also be seen. Acute renal failure and opportunistic infection such as candida are rare but have been reported.

The CT appearances of multiple hypodensities could indicate **multiple areas of ischaemic damage.** CT is poor at distinguishing acute from chronic infarction, but in a young patient, with a short history of being unwell without previous vascular history or known vascular risk factors, multiple acute events would be more likely than acute on chronic strokes. Involvement of both cerebral hemispheres suggests a cardioembolic source or vasculitis rather than large artery atherosclerosis (severe symptomatic carotid stenosis typically causes multiple lesions in the anterior circulation territory of a single hemisphere). An important cause of cardioembolic stroke, particularly in the young, is **infective endocarditis** (see page 150) and, given the presence of fever, systolic murmur and haematuria in this patient, infective endocarditis diagnosis must be excluded.

Vasculitis is another important cause of multiple strokes. This patient had a history of recently diagnosed asthma, facial rash, haematuria and relatively high ESR and low CRP. Asthma in combination with vasculitis suggests possible **Churg–Strauss syndrome** (see page 288) although renal involvement is unusual in this form of primary vasculitis and one would expect eosinophilia. CNS vasculitis occurs in Churg–Strauss (and the other forms of necrotising vasculitis such as polyarteritis nodosa) and causes encephalopathy with global cognitive decline and rarely strokes (see page 289). Alternatively, the presence of a butterfly rash together with low CRP but high ESR and haematuria could be consistent with **SLE**, which is associated with stroke. The aetiology of stroke in SLE is frequently attributed to vasculitis but in fact CNS vasculitis appears to be rare, whereas stroke secondary to cardioembolism from Libman–Sacks endocarditis, or to the presence of thrombogenic antibodies such as lupus anticoagulant, is much more common. About 75% of patients with SLE have CNS involvement at some point, often during the first year, the most common manifestation of which is psychosis or affective disorder. **Primary (isolated) CNS vasculitis** may cause encephalopathy and strokes (see page 174) and the CSF may be normal, but fever is not typical (present in around 15%) and by definition other organ systems are not affected so the haematuria in this case would have to be related to a separate pathological process.

Other inflammatory conditions such as **sarcoid** (see page 273) can cause fever, headache, encephalopathy and stroke-like episodes secondary to associated vasculitis or to space occupying lesions. Although skin lesions are common in sarcoid, the rash in this patient is not typical: sarcoid typically causes nodules and erythema nodosum. **ADEM** is an acute, uniphasic rapidly progressive central demyelinating disorder, often associated with viral infection (e.g. measles) or post-vaccination that is thought to be immune mediated (antibodies to the virus or to the vaccine cross-react with epitopes in the CNS cf paraneopolastic disorders). In some, but not all, there is a prodromal phase of fever, malaise and myalgia followed within a few days by encephalopathy and focal neurological signs. Peak deficit usually occurs within days and is followed by recovery over weeks to months. CSF usually shows elevated protein and mild pleocytosis but may be normal. Oligoclonal bands are usually absent. The diagnosis is often clear if there is a preceding history of a vaccine (e.g. rabies) or infection (e.g. measles) known to be strongly associated with ADEM. In other cases the differential diagnosis is broad as in the case described here. A severe first episode of MS may be difficult to distinguish from ADEM until the typical relapsing and remitting course of the disease emerges.

Other encephalopathies associated with stroke-like episodes include **Hashimoto's encephalitis** (see page 98) and **MELAS** (see page 103). White matter abnormalities have been reported on MRI with Hashimoto's encephalitis. MELAS typically causes cortical abnormalities, frequently in the parieto-occipital regions, that do not correspond to typical vascular boundaries. The features of this case were thus not typical of this condition. **CADASIL** (page 71) causes multiple strokes and chronic encephalopathy but one would not expect such an acute presentation, and the strokes are subcortical.

14c) The MRI scan shows multifocal white matter abnormalities leukoencephalopathy) seen particularly in the right cerebellum (Figs. 14.2a and 14.2b), and the right and left frontal regions (Figs. 14.3a and 14.3d, e respectively). The MRA (Fig. 18f) appears normal.

The differential diagnosis for these MRI findings is:
- Vasculitis
- PML
- ADEM

- Cytotoxic chemotherapy/radiation therapy

- Cardioembolic stroke.

There are many conditions that can cause a diffuse white matter abnormality or leukoencephalopathy. Some are rare inherited disorders, which will not be discussed further here. CT and MRI show non-specific

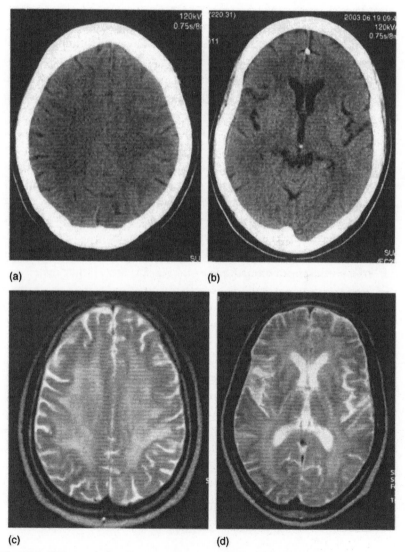

(a) (b)

(c) (d)

Fig. 14.3 HIV encephalopathy in a patient with advanced HIV infection: CT brain (a and b) shows widespread symmetrical confluent white matter hypodensity and cerebral atrophy seen more clearly on T2-weighted MRI (c and d).

abnormalities in isolated CNS vasculitis. CT is often normal but may show focal or multifocal low density areas. Association with haemorrhage or cortical atrophy suggests vasculitis. MRI shows non-specific T2-weighted hyperintensity without periventricular distribution, sometimes with leukoencephalopathy (a periventricular location suggests MS). The MRA may show beading of vessels but is usually normal owing to poor resolution for smaller vessels. In polyarteritis nodosa (PAN) (and Churg–Strauss), strokes are rare, but those that do occur are usually lacunar, frequently affecting the basal ganglia and internal capsule, although large artery stroke and haemorrhage may be seen. Diffuse multifocal white matter disease may occur in SLE and is often attributed to vasculitis. However, such changes are often the result of subacute infarcts and oedema. Brain biopsies frequently show multiple vessel occlusions with recanalization.

ADEM causes diffuse white matter abnormalities (periventricular and ovoid) on T2-weighted MRI, and often appears similar to MS in the early stages, but in ADEM, lesions resolve, at least partially, over weeks, without the appearance of new lesions. A first episode of MS may thus be clinically difficult to distinguish from ADEM. In the case of the current patient, the MRI lesions are not seen in the periventricular region typical of MS.

Sarcoid can cause diffuse T2-weighted hyperintensity.

Focal or multifocal well-defined, asymmetrical lesions without contrast enhancement or mass effect occur in subcortical white matter and sometimes the cerebellum, brainstem and spinal cord in progressive multifocal leukoencephalopathy (PML) (see below). In non-AIDS associated PML, early lesions tend to be in the subcortical white matter of the occipital lobes.

Similar leukoencephalopathic appearances may be seen following CNS radiation therapy or treatment with intrathecal methotrexate or other cytotoxic agents that cause demyelination. CT shows white matter hypodensity, cortical atrophy, and ventricular enlargement. MRI shows T2-weighted hyperintensity extending from the ventricles to the corticomedullary junction.

14d) The differential diagnoses following the MRI scan includes:

- Vasculitis:
  - Primary (isolated) CNS vasculitis
  - Secondary vasculitis.
- Immunodeficiency related:
  - PML.

The MRI findings showing multifocal white matter abnormality together with the clinical features narrow the differential diagnosis a little. **Vasculitis** remains in the differential diagnosis of which isolated (primary) CNS vasculitis (see page 174) would be high on the list. PAN/Churg–Strauss do not typically cause diffuse white matter abnormality but such changes may be seen with SLE.

The presence of oral candida in this patient suggests underlying immunodeficiency. **PML** is an opportunistic infection (probable virus reactivation) with the JC virus, which causes subacute demyelination of the CNS. It is associated with advanced HIV infection, and other disorders of cell-mediated immunity e.g. sarcoid, TB, lymphoproliferative disorders, and prolonged immunosuppression. The incidence has risen since the 1980s because of the association with AIDS (85% of patients with PML have associated HIV infection). Asymmetrical abnormalities of CNS white matter occur causing focal deficits. Motor weakness, behavioural change, cognitive impairment, cerebellar ataxia, and sensory abnormalities, are frequent. Headache, seizures and extrapyramidal features are rare. Onset is usually subacute and fever is infrequent, and there is progression to dementia as the number of lesions increases. CSF is usually normal. Brain biopsy shows unique abnormalities with oligonucleocytes containing enlarged nuclei with inclusion bodies and viral particles. JC viral DNA may be detected in CSF using PCR.

HIV dementia can cause neuroradiological findings similar to PML with ill-defined symmetrical (in contrast to the well-defined asymmetrical abnormalities usually seen in PML) T2–weighted abnormalities in white matter and atrophy (see Fig. 14.3).

HIV dementia is characterised by the presence of global cognitive dysfunction without the characteristic focal features seen in PML unless there is another neurological disorder present. HIV dementia occurs in advanced HIV infection usually in patients known to have AIDS. The features resemble a subcortical dementia with apathy, mental slowing, impaired concentration and memory. Motor signs include slowed rapid limb movements, gait disorder and spasticity. Early stages may resemble depression. Stroke is increased in patients with HIV infection and the causes are multiple but include vasculitis, either caused by the virus itself or as a result of opportunistic infection (e.g. aspergillus), syphilis, and VZV. **HIV seroconversion** is associated with a variety of neurological syndromes (see page 264) including acute CNS demyelinating disorders and needs to be excluded.

This patient's partner admitted to having being diagnosed as HIV positive 1 year earlier but had not told the patient about his diagnosis. This patient's HIV test was positive and the CD_4 count was low with reversal of the normal CD_4/CD_8 ratio (100 cells/mm^3 (8%) vs 980 cells/mm^3 (78%) for CD4 and CD8 cells respectively).

Further reading

Berger JR, Levy RM (eds) (1997). *AIDS and the nervous system* (2nd ed). Philadelphia: Lippincott-Raven.

Boska MD, Mosley RL, Nawab M *et al* (2004). Advances in neuroimaging for HIV-1 associated neurological dysfunction: clues to the diagnosis, pathogenesis and therapeutic monitoring. *Curr HIV Res*; 2(1):61–78. Review.

Koralnik IJ (2004). New insights into progressive multifocal leukoencephalopathy. *Curr Opin Neurol*; 17(3):365–70. Review.

Von Einsiedel RW, Fife TD, Aksamit AJ *et al* (1993). Progressive multifocal leukoencephalopathy in AIDS: a clinicopathologic study and review of the literature. *J Neurol*; 240(7):391–406.

Case 15

Case A A 40-year-old travel agent was referred with possible Guillain–Barré syndrome. He complained of a 2-week history of paraesthesia affecting the right inner thigh and spreading down to the right leg. Five days previously, he had developed pins and needles around the left ankle spreading upwards to the left groin and buttocks. He had been unable to sleep because of the painful sensation of the bedclothes on his legs. Two days prior to admission he had developed headache, nausea and left facial weakness. There was no past medical history of note, he was a non-smoker, took moderate alcohol, and was married with 2 children. He had recently returned from holiday. He had been taking paracetamol but no other medication.

On examination, he was well, apyrexial and general systems were unremarkable. There was no neck stiffness but there was a left lower motor neuron VII weakness. Examination of the upper limbs was normal. Lower limb power was normal but pin prick and temperature sensation was subjectively reduced behind the right knee and over the lateral aspect of the right calf. Lower limb reflexes were brisk and plantar reflexes were downgoing.

Investigations showed:

- Hb 16g/dL, WCC 9.9×10^9/L, plt 313×10^9/L, ESR 10mm/h
- U&E, LFT, glc, Ca all normal. Rh F <20, ANA negative. CXR normal
- CSF: opening pressure 20cm H_2O, RBC 8mm^3, WCC 688mm^3 (poly-morphs 6, lymphocytes 682), glc 2.5mmol/L (serum 7.9mmol/L), protein 2.0g/L, no organisms seen
- Viral PCR screen negative, cryptococcal ag negative, no oligoclonal bands
- NCS: normal sensory and motor conduction, f waves were absent in right common peroneal nerve.

Case B A 43-year-old man developed low back pain playing golf. Two weeks later this had worsened and he had a burning band around his waist, which radiated down to his thighs on standing. By the following month he noticed reduced appetite, one stone weight loss, night sweats, occasional twitches in his arms and legs, and a tremor in his hands. He was working as an accountant, smoked 25 cigarettes a day, and drank little alcohol. He was not on any medication.

On examination, general systems were normal and he was apyrexial. There was a postural tremor in the hands. The nervous system was unremarkable except for an absent ankle jerk on the left and an upgoing left plantar.

Investigations showed:

- FBC, ESR, U&E, glucose, LFT, Ca, TFT, CRP, B12, immunoglobulins, serum electrophoresis,CMV, EBV, autoantibody screen: all normal
- CXR: normal
- Nerve conduction studies: unremarkable
- MRI brain: normal
- MRI cord is shown in Fig. 15.1.

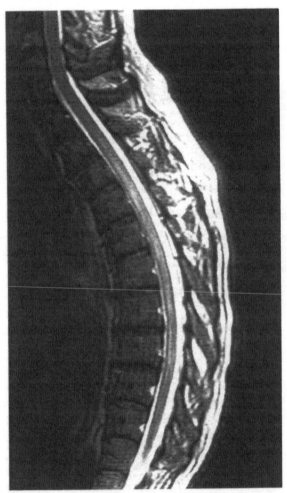

Fig. 15.1 Sagittal T2-weighted MRI spine from case A): in the upper thoracic cord, signal is normal, but in the mid thoracic cord there is pathological high signal over several segments without cord swelling.

- LP: CSF: WCC 182/mm^3 (174 lymphocytes, 8 polymorphs), protein 1.9g/L, glucose 2.8mmol/L (blood glucose 7.9mmol/L). Cytology was reported as 'lymphoma'
- CT thorax and abdomen and bone marrow: unremarkable.

One month after presentation, he was significantly improved and back playing golf. Repeat CSF showed a reduction in pleocytosis and protein level.

Case C A 52-year-old man developed fever, malaise and arthralgia. One week later he noticed right facial weakness and difficulty closing the right eye. Two days after this, the left eye became difficult to close and he self referred to the emergency department.

On examination, he was apyrexial, and general systems were normal. Neurological examination revealed bilateral VII nerve palsies.

Questions

15a) Give three conditions associated with bilateral lower motor neuron palsy.

15b) Where are the lesions causing the sensory symptoms in cases A and B?

15c) What is the most likely diagnosis applicable to all three cases?

15d) What further questions would you like to ask these patients? What is the virtually pathognomic symptom/sign that may or may not be present?

15e) Describe the clinical features of this condition with particular reference to the neurological abnormalities that may occur.

Answers

15a) Bilateral VII nerve palsy occurs in:

- Lyme disease
- Sarcoid
- Guillain–Barré syndrome
- HIV.

The MRI from case C) is shown in Fig. 15.2 Bilateral facial weakness caused by myasthaenia gravis may mimic a bilateral VII nerve palsy. Although there are numerous other causes of lower motor neuron VII palsy (see page 284), bilateral abnormalities are rare.

15b) The lesions are in the:

- Spinal cord or brain (case A)
- Nerve roots (case B).

In case A, there is patchy distal dysaesthesia and objective sensory signs that do not correspond with a dermatomal or peripheral nerve distribution and thus may have a central origin. In case B, the symptoms of a band like pain round the thorax suggests a radiculopathy affecting thoracic nerve roots. The extension of pain on standing suggests mechanical stretch of nerve routes supplying the trunk and thighs or inflammation of the cord carrying impulses from this area of the periphery (cf. Lhermitte's phenomenon).

15c) The most likely diagnosis is **Lyme disease**.

Taken together, these cases show VII cranial neuropathy (bilateral in case C), radiculopathy and myelopathy and/or peripheral neuropathy

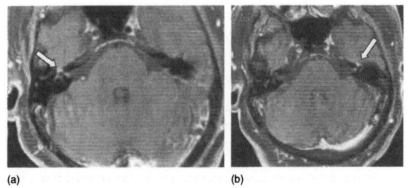

(a)   (b)

Fig. 15.2 Contrast enhanced axial MRI showing bilateral facial nerve enhancement (geniculate ganglion, arrows) in the patient from case C.

with associated features of an inflammatory disorder in cases B and C. The most likely diagnosis is Lyme disease caused by the spirochaete *Borrelia burgdorferi* and closely related strains.

HIV seroconversion (see page 263) is a possible alternative diagnosis since this may cause bilateral VII nerve palsy, peripheral neuropathy/radiculopathy, and non specific symptoms consistent with an inflammatory disorder. There were no features to support a diagnosis of **sarcoid** although isolated neurological disease may occur. **Guillain–Barré** syndrome (see page 76) would not explain the clinical features seen in all 3 cases and the CSF in Guillain–Barré syndrome is usually acellular.

15d) Patients should be asked about outdoor activities and prior history of rash. Erythema migrans is the pathognomic sign.

Lyme disease is transmitted by tick bites and is therefore more likely to occur following outdoor activities (e.g. camping, walking in endemic areas), and patients should be asked about such activities and the possibility of tick bites in the preceding few weeks. Lyme disease typically begins with a virtually pathognomic rash, erythema migrans (erythema chronicum migrans) (see below) occurring at the site of the tick bite. Between one half to two thirds of adults recall having a rash. The patient described in case A had been camping in a deer park two months prior to presentation followed 4 weeks later by a skin lesion behind the right knee that had a black centre and red surround. This lesion had expanded over a few days before disappearing.

15e) The clinical features include:

- Rash
- Fever
- Lymphadenopathy
- Arthralgia
- Heart block
- Central and peripheral nervous system abnormalities.

Lyme disease is more common in the warmer months (spring to autumn) as this is when the ticks feed. Different strains of the bacterium are present in Europe (e.g. *B. burgdorferi garinii* and *B. burgdorferi afzelii*) and the USA (*B. burgdorferi sensu stricto*) resulting in different frequencies of the various clinical features seen in patients from the two continents. In Europe, skin lesions are often single, there is arthralgia rather than arthritis, and meningeal symptoms may be absent whereas radiculitis may be prominent and accompanied by severe pain. Progressive encephalomyelitis is a late complication. Arthritis and meningitis are more common in the USA form with later encephalopathy being more common than the more severe encephalomyelitis.

The first phase of the disease is local infection characterized by erythema migrans which occurs within one month of the tick bite and may be itchy and burning. The rash contains many spirochaetes especially at its leading edge. The rash expands outwards from the centre, which is usually erythematous and indurated but may be necrotic, occasionally to cover a whole limb or the trunk. As the rash enlarges peripherally, the centre clears. The second phase of the disease is early dissemination of spirochaetes associated with systemic upset, fever, arthralgias, myalgias and lymphadenopathy without gastrointestinal or respiratory involvement. The third phase is of more chronic dissemination associated with relapsing and remitting symptoms that may include arthritis, radiculoneuritis, encephalitis, and cardiac dysfunction. About 5% of patients develop cardiac abnormalities typically heart block. Arthritis may begin months after disease onset and commonly affects the knee, although both large and small joints may be affected. In 10% of cases, arthritis may become chronic and erosive.

Around 10–15% of patients develop neurological abnormalities, which may include the following:

- Meningitis
- Encephalitis/encephalopathy
- Localized CNS vasculitis
- Cranial neuropathy
- Transverse myelitis
- Radiculitis
- Peripheral (axonal) neuropathy (diffuse polyneuropathy or mononeuritis multiplex)
- Inflammatory myopathy.

Neurological abnormalities may be caused directly by nervous system infection (e.g. encephalomyelitis) or indirectly by immune (parainfectious) mechanisms (e.g. mild encephalopathy). In lymphocytic meningitis, the degree of headache and neck stiffness is variable and although the illness occurs acutely, occasionally a relapsing and remitting course may be seen together with obstructive hydrocephalus. Typically the CSF contains from 50 to several hundred cells/mm^3 with mild protein elevation and glucose is usually normal. Although culture of *B. burgdorferi* is possible, fewer than 10% of patients have positive CSF culture probably owing to the low concentration of organisms in the CSF. Although reactive meningitis is common, encephalomyelitis is rare and usually associated with greater levels of pleocytosis and MR imaging abnormalities principally affecting the white matter. Focal deficits may occur but the prognosis with treatment is good. There are a few reports of stroke associated with Lyme disease possibly secondary to vasculitis.

The cranial nerves are often affected in Lyme disease. As in syphilis and other forms of basilar meningitis, cranial nerves VII and VIII are most commonly involved although abnormalities of III–VI may also be seen. Involvement of the lower cranial nerves and the optic nerve is rare. Lyme disease is one of the few disorders, along with sarcoid, HIV and Guillain–Barré syndrome, commonly associated with bilateral VII nerve palsies (see earlier), so patients presenting with bilateral VII nerve palsies, particularly in endemic areas, should undergo serological testing for Lyme disease.

The peripheral nervous system is involved probably more frequently than the CNS. Severe radicular pain may mimic mechanical radiculopathy and nocturnal pain may be severe. Weakness in the nerve root distribution may be minimal or severe. Radiculoneuritis may continue for months after initial infection. The CSF is often normal if the CNS is not involved. Diffuse non-painful distal polyneuropathy with sensorimotor involvement is also common. Mononeuritis multiplex and plexopathies may occur. There are a few reports of a Guillain–Barré-like syndrome but pleocytosis is more common in Lyme disease than typically occurs with GBS and electrophysiological studies do not generally show demyelination.

Some later manifestations of neurological involvement in Lyme disease are controversial. Encephalopathy with cognitive abnormalities, accelerated dementia with normal CSF, have been reported. Other psychiatric and fatigue syndromes appear less likely to be directly related.

Treatment regimens vary according to the clinical features present. Erythema migrans should be treated immediately with oral medication (doxycycline or amoxicillin). CNS involvement is treated with intravenous third generation cephalosporins although optimal duration of treatment is unclear and most patients receive at least 2 weeks of therapy.

Further reading

Haass A (1998). Lyme neuroborreliosis. *Curr Opin Neurol*; 11(3):253–258.

Halperin JJ (2003). Lyme disease and the peripheral nervous system. *Muscle Nerve*; 28(2):133–143.

Halperin JJ (2003). Facial nerve palsy associated with Lyme disease. *Muscle Nerve*; 28(4):516–7.

Steere AC, Sikand VK (2003). The presenting manifestations of Lyme disease and the outcomes of treatment. *New Engl J Med*; 348(24):2472–2474.

Case 16

A 34-year-old woman was admitted for urgent investigation of twitching of the face and jerking of the legs and arms that had begun 3 weeks earlier. On one occasion, her right arm had jerked when she was holding a glass of water, causing her to drop it. Over the preceding 2 years, she had had multiple episodes of stuttering speech and slight mental slowing lasting for days to several weeks, during which she had found it difficult to function at work. On 3 occasions, she had suffered a sudden loss of consciousness, and tonic clonic activity associated with prolactin rise was seen on one occasion. After each episode she had had a 'prolonged postictal period'. Cerebral MRI had been unremarkable. She had been prescribed carbamezepine. There was no other past medical history and she worked as a marketing manager.

On examination, there was a fine tremor of the outstretched hands. Occasional myoclonic jerks were seen in the face and fingers. There were no focal neurological abnormalities on examination and general systems were normal.

Investigations showed:

- FBC, U&E, LFT, CRP, ESR, complement, immunoglobulins, vasculitic screen: normal.
- Carbamezepine level: 35μmol/L (normal)
- MRI brain: unremarkable
- CSF examination including for oligoclonal bands: unremarkable
- EEG performed over a 4-day period with videotelemetry: paroxysms of delta slow wave activity over the fronto-temporal regions bilaterally. No epileptiform activity seen
- TSH 12.8mu/L (0.5–6.0mu/L), total thyroxine 55mmol/L (70–140mmol/L).

A further test was performed and she was started on steroids and thyroxine with good resolution of her symptoms. However, on reducing the steroids, she became shaky and tremulous with a sensation of unsteadiness. This resolved on increasing the steroid dose.

Questions

16a) What is the most likely diagnosis?

16b) What are the clinical features of this condition?

16c) How would you treat this patient?

Answers

16a) The most likely diagnosis is **Hashimoto's encephalitis.**

The diagnosis of Hashimoto's encephalitis is made on the basis of the clinical findings together with exclusion of other causes of encephalopathy and the presence of elevated thyroid antibody titres (see below). In this case, the relapsing and remitting course of the illness, myoclonus, stroke-like episodes and seizures were typical of Hashimoto's encephalitis. The mild hypothyroidism prompted measurement of thyroid peroxidase antibody which was elevated at 1388IU/ml (0–75IU/ml).

16b) Hashimoto's encephalopathy is seen in patients with elevated thyroid autoantibodies and is more common in females.

An association between Hashimoto's thyroiditis and encephalopathy was first suggested by Brain in 1966. It has no specific clinical features and therefore other causes of encephalopathy including infectious, metabolic, toxic, inflammatory, neoplastic, paraneoplastic, and vascular diseases, should be excluded. Alteration in thyroid metabolic status does not explain the encephalopathy since the majority of patients are euthyroid at presentation, and those who are hypothyroid initially may relapse on thyroxine therapy when euthyroid, as seen in this patient.

Confusion and reduction in conscious level may be abrupt in onset or there may be insidious cognitive decline. Seizures are common. A relapsing and remitting course, associated tremor and/or myoclonus and episodes of stroke-like deterioration are characteristic. The CSF protein is usually elevated without a pleocytosis and antithyroid antibody may be detected. EEG shows generalized or focal slow wave activity. Brain imaging is usually normal although white matter abnormalities have been reported, in one case apparently resolving with steroid treatment.

The mechanism of Hashimoto's encephalopathy is unknown and no systematic histopathological examinations have been carried out. Immune complex deposition with an associated vasculitis has been proposed. This is supported by the occasional association with immune complex glomerulonephritis and vasculitic neuropathy. It is not thought that the antithyroid antibodies themselves are pathogenic and there is no correlation between the level or type of antibody and the severity or clinical features of the encephalopathy.

16c) Hashimoto's encephalopathy is treated with immunosuppression.

Hashimoto's encephalopathy responds well to steroids although occasionally additional immunosuppressant therapy may be required. The outlook with treatment is generally good with complete remission rates of 80–96%. As seen in this case, relapse may occur off steroids with symptoms responding rapidly to reintroduction of treatment.

Further reading

Chong JY, Rowland LP and Utiger RD (2003). Hashimoto encephalopathy: syndrome or myth? *Arch Neurol*; **60**(2):164–171.

Ghika-Schmid F, Ghika J, Regli F *et al* (1996). Hashimoto's myoclonic encephalopathy: an underdiagnosed treatable condition? *Mov Disord*; **11**:555–562.

Kothbauer-Margreiter I, Sturzenegger M, *et al* (1996). Encephalopathy associated with Hashimoto thyroiditis: diagnosis and treatment. *J Neurol*; **243**(8):585–593.

Shaw PJ, Walls TJ, Newman PK *et al* (1991). Hashimoto's encephalopathy: a steroid-responsive disorder associated with high anti-thyroid antibody titers–report of 5 cases. *Neurology*; **41**(2):228–233.

Case 17

A 40-year-old man developed sudden-onset speech difficulty whilst at work and the following day became increasingly confused. He was seen by his GP later that day who found that he was unable to follow commands. There was no history of associated headache, fever, or weakness. There was no family history or past medical history of note. The patient was not taking any medication and denied illicit drug use.

On examination, the patient was apyrexial, thin, confused, and agitated. The neck was not stiff. There was both expressive and receptive aphasia. Cranial nerves were normal with the exception of the presence of a hearing aid. The fundi could not be seen owing to lack of patient co-operation. The upper limbs were wasted proximally with increased tone on the right and although all 4 limbs were moving, the right appeared dyspraxic and the patient favoured the left. Lower limb power appeared full, reflexes were brisk and symmetrical and the right plantar was equivocal. Shortly after admission, the patient suffered two *grand mal* seizures.

Investigations showed:

- FBC, U&E, LFT, TSH, CK: normal
- CRP 51mg/L, fasting glucose 6.3mm/L
- ANCA and ANA: negative
- CSF: acellular, protein 1.2g/L, glucose 3.9mm/L, no organisms
- EEG: slow wave activity in the left temporal and occipital lobes.

CT and MRI brain scans are shown in Fig. 17.1 and 17.2 respectively.

Questions

17a) Give the differential diagnosis you would have considered before obtaining the investigation results.

17b) What does the brain imaging show?

17c) Which is the most likely diagnosis?

17d) What are the clinical features of this condition?

17e) What investigations would help in diagnosis?

17f) Is there a definitive diagnostic test?

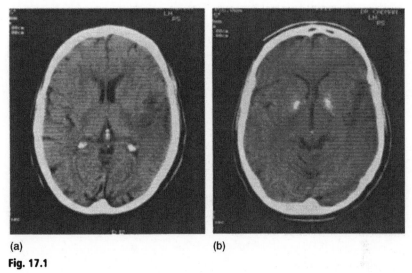

(a)   (b)

Fig. 17.1

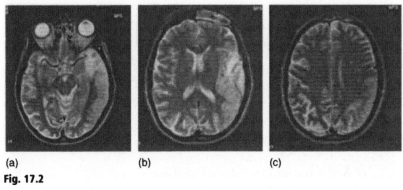

(a)   (b)   (c)

Fig. 17.2

Answers

17a) The differential diagnosis in this case is wide and, depending on the significance placed on the apparent wasting of the proximal upper limb muscles, could include any of the following disorders:

- Vascular:
  - Stroke
  - Venous sinus thrombosis (see page 10)
  - Subdural haematoma.
- Infectious:
  - HSV (see page 6), *HIV* (see page 263)
  - TB (see page 54)
  - Cryptococcus (see page 42), aspergillus
  - Toxoplasma
  - Cerebral abscess
  - Whipple's disease.
- Inflammatory:
  - *Sarcoid* (see page 273)
  - *Connective tissue disease*
  - Acute disseminated encephalomyelitis (ADEM)
  - Vasculitis (see page 174)
  - Hashimoto's encephalitis (see page 98).
- Metabolic:
  - Hypoglycaemia
  - Electrolyte disturbance (see page 136)
  - *Mitochondrial disease.*
- Neoplastic:
  - Space occupying lesion, *paraneoplastic syndrome* (see page 252).

Diagnoses in italics indicate those in which there is the possibility of an associated proximal myopathy.

The clinical features of this case indicate a stroke-like episode (sudden onset of speech difficulty) followed by encephalopathy (confusion). The stroke-like episode suggests a vascular aetiology but other non vascular disorders may present with sudden onset focal deficits and should be considered where there are atypical clinical features, such as an absence of vascular risk factors, or unusual imaging findings.

17b) The CT brain shows basal ganglia calcification and a hypodense region in the left temporal lobe. The T2-weighted MRI brain shows a primarily cortical hyperintensity in the left temporal parietal region not typical of a middle cerebral artery branch infarction.

17c) The diagnosis is **mitochodrial encephalopathy, lactic acidosis, and stroke-like episodes (MELAS).**

17d) MELAS should always be considered in any young to middle-aged patient with a stroke in the absence of any other obvious cause, particularly if the stroke is in the occipital region and is associated with seizures.

MELAS is one of the multisystem disorders associated with mutations of mitochondrial DNA inherited through the maternal line. Mitochondrial DNA encodes proteins involved in the respiratory chain. The phenotypes of the various mitochondrial diseases are characteristic but often overlap. Cardiomyopathy, proximal muscle weakness (as in this case), progressive external opthalmoplegia, myoclonus, ataxia, exercise intolerance, pigmented retinopathy, and ovarian and testicular failure, are typical features.

MELAS presents in childhood or young to middle-aged adults often with focal neurological episodes that usually affect the occipital lobes, and may be triggered by infection. Hemianopia, cortical blindness, hemiparesis and aphasia may occur. Sudden onset headache, episodic vomiting and seizures are common. Ultimately, the patient becomes demented and often cortically blind. Associated clinical features include short stature, sensorineural deafness, mitochondrial myopathy, migraine, diabetes mellitus, peripheral neuropathy, learning disability, and salt and pepper retinopathy. Owing to phenotypic and genotypic heterogeneity, relatives of an index patient may not present with MELAS but rather with one of the other mitochondrial syndromes. The cause of the acute focal cerebral dysfunction is unclear but large vessel occlusion does not occur. Metabolic defects and structural changes in small vessels have been proposed.

17e) The following investigations are useful in diagnosis:

- Blood and CSF lactate levels
- Muscle biopsy
- Brain imaging.

Blood and CSF lactate levels are often increased as seen in this patient [3.3mm/L (normal range 0.5–2.0mmol/L) and 6.5mmol/L (normal <2.5mmol/L) respectively] owing to dysfunction of the respiratory chain, but similarly elevated CSF lactate levels may be seen after acute stroke of other aetiology, seizures, meningitis, and subarachnoid haemorrhage. Serum CK is often normal. Muscle biopsy usually shows a mitochondrial myopathy with ragged red fibres shown using Gomori's trichrome stain and large numbers of abnormal mitochondria on electron microscopy, although the latter may be normal.

Brain imaging shows basal ganglia calcification (as seen in this patient) in 50% of cases, always involving the globus pallidus. CT may show low density areas in the grey and white matter mainly in the occipital and parietal lobes and cerebellum with enhancement and mass effect in the acute phase. T2-weighted hyperintensities in the cortex are seen on MRI which may disappear on subsequent scans. Cerebral and cerebellar atrophy are seen and fourth ventricular enlargement may occur early. The lesions visible on brain imaging are often described as infarcts but do not correspond to the territories of the main cerebral arteries.

The diagnosis of MELAS can be confirmed by mitochondrial DNA analysis of white cells or skeletal muscle. A mitochondrial DNA point mutation at position 3243 within the tRNA$^{Leu(URR)}$ encoding gene is most commonly seen. This mutation is always heteroplasmic in that wild type DNA is also present, suggesting that wild type DNA is required for foetal viability. However, not all patients have known mutations and some of the known mutations may be found in patients with other mitochondrial syndromes. Further, relatives who carry the mutation may be asymptomatic and mutations can be found in the normal population.

Further reading

DiMauro S, Moraes CT (1993). Mitochondrial encephalomyopathies. *Arch Neurol*; 50(11):1197–1208.

Goto Y, Horai S, Matsuola T *et al* (1992). Mitochodrial encepthalopathy, lactic acidosis and stroke-like episodes (MELAS): a correlative study of the clinical features and mitochondrial DNA mutation. *Neurology*; 42(3,1):545–50.

Schmiedel J, Jackson S, Schafe S *et al* (2003). Mitochondrial cytopathies. *J Neurol*; 250(3):267–277.

Yilmaz EY, Love BB and Biller J (2001). Metabolic causes of stroke (pp 280–282) and Hirt L and Bogousslavsky J (2001). MELAS and stroke in mitochondrial diseases (pp 324–327) in: *Uncommon causes of stroke*. Bogousslavsky J and Caplan LR (eds). Cambridge University Press.

Case 18

A 63-year-old man presented with central crushing chest pain and was given thrombolysis for inferior myocardial infarction. He was not on any medication prior to admission, and aspirin, simvastatin, ramipril, spironolactone, carvedilol, and frusemide were started. There was a family history of premature coronary vascular disease. Three days following admission, he had a further myocardial infarct and received thrombolysis with tPA, after which he had a brief cardiac arrest followed by cardiogenic shock requiring dobutamine ionotropic support. Cardiac catheterization showed triple vessel disease requiring future cardiac bypass surgery.

The day after coronary catheterization, he noticed painful arms, and left arm and leg weakness. A CT brain showed no abnormality. The next day, he developed weakness of the right arm and leg associated with generalized aching in the limbs. His symptoms progressed such that 4 days later he was unable to walk or to lift his arms above his head. Bladder and bowel function remained normal. There was no neck or back pain. On examination, the cranial nerves were normal. Limb tone was unremarkable and there was no wasting but there was generalized muscle tenderness. There was severe proximal symmetrical limb weakness with relative preservation of distal power. The reflexes were normal and the plantar reflexes were downgoing. There was no sensory abnormality.

FBC, U&E, TFT, and Ca were normal.

Questions

18a) Which anatomical component of the patient's neuromuscular system is affected?

18b) List the causes of this type of lesion (acquired rather than congenital).

18c) What blood test would you like to perform? What else would you like to examine at the bedside?

18d) What is the most likely diagnosis? How would you confirm it?

18e) How would you treat this patient?

Answers

18a) The muscles have been affected.

A myopathy should be suspected in any patient presenting with symmetrical proximal limb weakness. Patients may complain of difficulty getting out of a chair, climbing stairs, or in combing/washing their hair. The major clinical sign is muscle weakness, and muscle wasting; hypotonia and decreased reflexes are usually only seen in advanced cases. Myalgia and cramps may or may not be present. CK may be elevated reflecting disruption to muscle fibre membranes. The EMG is often abnormal and muscle biopsy may be required for diagnosis.

An **acute neuropathy** (e.g. Guillain–Barré syndrome, porphyria, critical illness neuropathy) may be difficult to distinguish from an acute myopathy, particularly in the early stages when the reflexes may be preserved (see page 77). **Porphyria** (see page 65) may cause proximal weakness but this would not be expected in critical illness neuropathy, and there is often bilateral facial weakness and sensory symptoms in **Guillain–Barré** syndrome (see page 76). **Myasthenic crisis**, which may be precipitated by intercurrent illness or administration of certain drugs, may present with subacute limb weakness, but extra-ocular muscle weakness and ptosis are usually prominent, and there is often respiratory compromise.

The onset of symptoms after myocardial infarction, thrombolysis and cardiac catheterization in this patient, might lead one to suspect a vascular cause for his symptoms. **Brainstem ischaemia** may cause bilateral limb weakness and may have a stuttering onset (see page 28), but one would expect cranial nerve signs and signs consistent with an upper motor neuron lesion in the limbs. **Infarction of the cord** (e.g. after occlusion of the anterior spinal artery, see page 192) causes bilateral limb weakness but again one would expect upper motor neuron symptoms in the limbs after the acute phase.

18b) There are many causes of an acquired myopathy:

- *Endocrine:*
  - Hyper/hypothyroidism (see pages 35 and 124)
  - Acromegaly
  - Hyperparathyroidism
  - Osteomalacia
  - Cushing's disease.
- *Infectious:*
  - Pyogenic myositis (this causes focal rather then generalized symptoms and signs) e.g. *Staphylococcal aureus*

- Viruses e.g. influenza, adenovirus, influenza, CMV, EBV, HIV
- Fungal e.g. *Cryptococcus neoformans*
- Protozoa e.g. toxoplasma.

- *Inflammatory:*
  - Dermatomyositis, polymyositis, inclusion body myositis, sarcoid
  - Polymyalgia rheumatica (not strictly a myopathy — power is often reduced proximally secondary to pain).

- *Drugs:*
  - Steroids
  - Statins
  - Fibric acid derivatives
    and many others .

- *Toxic*
  - Hypokalaemia
  - Critical illness
  - Chronic renal failure
  - Alcohol.

Most of the endocrine associated myopathies are insidious and many patients remain asymptomatic. However, rarely symptoms may be florid and be the presenting feature of the illness. Hypo- and hyperthyroid-associated myopathies are discussed further, on pages 35 and 124 respectively. Briefly, in hypothyroidism, there is pain, stiffness and weakness in the proximal muscles which may mimic polymyalgia rheumatica, and CK is nearly always elevated. Exceptionally, severe, subacute myopathy may cause rhabdomyolysis and respiratory failure. Hyperthyroidism causes muscle weakness with proximal wasting and appears to be more common in men. It is apparent on clinical examination in the majority of patients. As in hypothyroid-associated myopathy, patients complain of difficulty with climbing stairs, getting out of a chair, or combing the hair. Occasionally, bulbar dysfunction, of which dysphagia is the most common feature, may occur with aspiration pneumonia. Rarely, ventilatory support may be necessary. Acute thyrotoxic myopathy has been described in which rapidly progressive symptoms caused severe weakness including of bulbar and respiratory muscles over days (although it is likely that many of these cases had coexistent myasthenia gravis). Reflexes may be reduced or absent but sphincter function is preserved. In contrast to hypothyroid myopathy, the CK is usually within the normal range but may be elevated in thyrotoxic crisis with rhabdomyolysis.

Thyrotoxic periodic paralysis is relatively common as a complication of hyperthyroidism in Asian populations, but is rare in other ethnic groups. Attacks are associated with a fall in the serum potassium and are identical to those seen in familial forms of hypokalaemic periodic paralysis with rapid onset recurrent flaccid weakness, predominantly of the proximal muscles and affecting the lower more then the upper limbs that may be heralded by cramps, aches or stiffness. Bulbar, ocular and respiratory muscles are usually spared. Attacks only occur when the patient is hyperthyroid and are most common in Graves' disease.

Exogenous or endogenous steroids are a common and thus important cause of myopathy in which there is selective atrophy of type II muscle fibres without necrosis or inflammation. The CK is usually normal. EMG does not show fibrillation potentials or sharp waves in contrast to the inflammatory myopathies (see page 22). Acromegaly causes slowly progressive weakness without wasting. There is mild elevation of the CK. Primary and secondary hyperparathyroidism occasionally cause a chronic myopathy in which the CK is normal.

Various infections are associated with myopathy. HIV causes a polymyositis-like syndrome (see pages 23 and 263), nemaline myopathy, type II muscle fibre atrophy and wasting syndrome, myoglobinuria, and pyomyositis. Acute myositis may be caused by a number of viruses including influenza, Coxsackie (Bornholm disease), EBV, CMV. Myalgia is the most common symptom but elevation of CK, rhabdomyolysis and myoglobinuria may occur. Toxoplasmosis, and several other protozoal infections, cause myositis, that associated with Toxoplasma being very similar to polymyositis. The inflammatory myopathies (dermatomyositis, polymyositis and inclusion body myositis) (see page 22) are usually subacute or chronic but may present acutely (dermatomyositis and polymyositis) and cause bulbar and respiratory muscle dysfunction. The CK level is usually elevated more in acute rather then chronic presentations of dermatomyositis or polymyositis (but may be normal in acute disease) and is modestly raised in inclusion body myositis.

Sarcoid causes granulomatous inflammation of muscle in around half of patients but most patients are asymptomatic. Fibrosis and palpable nodules in the muscles may occur and rarely there may be a myositis. Polymyalgia rheumatica causes myalgia and apparent mild weakness secondary to pain, in contrast to dermatomyositis and polymyositis, in which weakness rather than pain predominates. There are often systemic symptoms, raised ESR and anaemia and minor non specific abnormalities are seen on muscle biopsy.

Many different medications can cause a myopathy that may be acute beginning within weeks of introduction of the offending medication. CK may or may not (for example in steroid associated myopathy (see above)) be elevated. Critical illness can cause a necrotizing or non-necrotizing myopathy. Acute quadriplegic myopathy may occur in association with high dose steroids and neuromuscular blocking agents in which there is loss of the thick (myosin) filaments. CK is often normal. Weakness is often discovered when the patient is found to be ventilator-dependent. Differentiation from critical illness neuropathy may be difficult and some clinicians use the term neuromyopathy.

Alcohol causes a necrotising myopathy, usually in the context of chronic excess alcohol consumption. There is pain, proximal weakness, muscle swelling and tenderness, and in severe cases myoglobinuria may occur. The CK is elevated and there is muscle fibre necrosis. Occasionally, there may be a more insidious onset of symptoms without myalgia. The CK is normal and there are no fibrillation potentials or positive sharp waves. Muscle biopsy reveals atrophy of type II fibres. Uraemia causes a similar picture to chronic alcoholic myopathy and hyper-parathyroidism and may be caused by secondary hyperparathyroidism. Hypokalaemia causes proximal weakness, associated with myoglobinuria and CK elevation in severe cases. Potassium replacement leads to rapid improvement.

18c) CK should be requested together with inspection and laboratory testing of the urine for myoglobinuria.

In this patient, the CK was >42 000IU/L (normal range 25–195IU/L) and the urine was dark brown secondary to myoglobin.

18d) The most likely diagnosis is simvastatin-associated myopathy (in actual fact simvastatin-induced rhabdomyolysis as shown by the very high CK level and myoglobinuria).

Diagnosis can be confirmed on muscle biopsy which shows an acute necrotic myopathy consistent with statin induced disease. The pathological features are not specific but helps exclude other disorders such as myositis.

This patient has developed a rapidly progressive myopathy since coming into hospital. This suggests an iatrogenic cause, most likely drug-related. **Drug-related myopathy** is an important diagnosis to make as patients usually recover well if medication is stopped soon enough but may progress to rhabdomyolysis and death from renal failure if the condition is not recognised. As with any adverse drug reaction, the causal relationship between the muscle disorder and the drug is suggested by:

- Lack of pre-existing muscle symptoms
- Presence of a reasonable temporal relationship between the start of treatment and the appearance of symptoms
- Lack of any other cause for the myopathy
- Partial or complete resolution of symptoms after the toxic agent is withdrawn.

Acute myositis (see page 22) should be included in the differential diagnosis in this patient with a history of Raynaud's phenomenon since myositis occurs frequently in association with underlying rheumatological disease, such as SLE or rheumatoid arthritis. Investigations show no evidence of an endocrine abnormality that could explain his symptoms and there is nothing to suggest infection. Critical illness myopathy usually occurs in the context of ITU admission.

Simvastatin, one of the HMG CoA reductase inhibitor class of drugs (statins), is well known to cause myopathy. Drug induced myopathy may be acute or subacute and symptoms begin days or weeks after starting medication. There is a broad clinical spectrum of **statin-associated myopathy** from mild muscle aches to severe muscle pain and restriction in mobility which can be divided into four syndromes:

- Myositis/rhabdomyolysis (0.15 deaths per million prescriptions)
- Asymptomatic CK elevation
- Myalgia and muscle weakness(1–5% in trials, similar to placebo) usually with elevated CK. Symptoms may persist after statin withdrawal.
- Exercise-induced muscle pain not associated with weakness or CK elevation.

The risks are increased with increasing serum concentrations as a result of high doses or impaired metabolism, decreased renal/hepatic function, hypothyroidism, diabetes mellitus, concomitant medication including fibric acid derivatives, ciclosporin, macrolide antibiotics, HIV protease inhibitors, verapamil, diltiazem, amiodarone, and large amounts of grapefruit juice. Conditions predisposing to rhabdomyolysis (trauma, sepsis, drug abuse) also potentiate the myotoxicity of statins.

18e) Simvastatin should be stopped. Hydration should be maintained together with forced alkaline diuresis in this case.

Rhabdomyolysis causes myoglobinuria, as muscle breakdown releases myoglobin, a haeme-binding protein in muscle sarcoplasm that stores oxygen. The major complication of rhabdomyolysis is renal failure from myoglobin-induced renal tubular necrosis. Treatment is with forced alkaline diuresis, which this patient was given, and plasmapharesis in severe cases. The prognosis for complete recovery is excellent and this patient left hospital one month later with normal muscle power and normal CK.

Other causes of rhabdomyolysis are given below:

- Infection:
  - See myopathy list above.
- Drugs:
  - Neuroleptic malignant syndrome
  - Malignant hyperthermia secondary to anaesthetics.
- Metabolic derangement:
  - Hypokalaemia
  - DKA/HONC
  - Hyper/hypothyroidism.
- Overexertion:
  - Catatonic rigidity
  - Status epilepticus
  - Tetanus
  - Chorea
  - Acute pyschosis.
- Inflammatory myositis
- Toxins:
  - Snake/spider/fish/wasp/bee toxins
  - Cocaine/amphetamine/ecstasy
  - Alcohol.
- Trauma/infarction:
  - Crush injury
  - Compartment syndrome
  - Vascular occlusion.

Management of asymptomatic patients with CK elevation secondary to simvastatin is unclear. If the CK is elevated to less than 3–5 times normal, it has been suggested that the patient should be monitored and the drug withdrawn only if symptoms develop whereas greater levels of CK elevation should prompt cessation of therapy. In patients with myalgia in the absence of CK elevation, the drug should be stopped if symptoms are intolerable. An alternative drug of the same class can be introduced once the patient has become asymptomatic. Lower statin doses should be used in high risk patients.

Further reading

Argov Z (2000). Drug-induced myopathies. *Curr Opin Neurol*; 13:541–545.

Bannwarth B (2002). Drug-induced myopathies. Expert Opin. *Drug Saf*, 1(1):65–70.

Rosenson RS (2004). Current overview of statin-induced myopathy. *Am J Med*; 116(6):408–416.

Case 19

Case A A 60-year-old woman developed sudden onset pulsatile tinnitus in her left ear. Three weeks later she developed left-sided leg and arm weakness that resolved over 2 days. Two days later there was a recurrence of the left-sided weakness accompanied by dysarthria. On examination, there was a left carotid bruit and a right Horner's syndrome and mild left upper motor neuron face, and hand weakness. The rest of the neurological examination was normal.

Case B A 57-year-old man awoke with a pain behind his right eye. The eyelid looked swollen and shut but he was able to open it with his fingers, whereupon he noticed slight blurring and occasional double vision, and the eye looked red. The symptoms resolved over the next day but 3 days later he awoke with right sided pulsatile tinnitus, a puffy closed right eye, blurred and double vision and weakness and numbness of the left face, arm and leg, all of which resolved over a few hours. He was a smoker of 35 cigarettes a day.

On examination, he was normotensive with no bruits and in sinus rhythm with no murmurs but dorsalis pedis pulses were absent bilaterally. Pupillary responses and eye movements were normal but visual acuity was reduced to 6/9 in the right eye.

Questions

19a) What is the diagnosis that applies to both cases? Explain each patient's symptoms and signs.

19b) What abnormalities on radiological investigations might you expect to see?

19c) What are the clinicopathologic features of this condition?

19d) Which underlying medical disorders are associated with this condition?

19e) What specific points in the history and examination should be looked for?

19f) How would you treat these patients?

Answers

19a) The diagnosis in each case is **internal carotid artery dissection:**

Case A) bilateral internal carotid dissection

Case B) right internal carotid artery dissection

In case A, the left-sided pulsatile tinnitus suggests a left vascular abnormality. The sudden onset suggests a dissection. The left-sided weakness and dysarthria is consistent with an abnormality of the right motor cortex or the descending motor pathways on the right. The left carotid bruit suggests a left carotid abnormality and the right Horner's syndrome suggests a right carotid dissection with consequent right hemisphere ischaemia.

In case B, the development of right pulsatile tinnitus and left sided sensory symptoms is consistent with right carotid dissection and right hemisphere ischaemic stroke. The associated pain and ptosis of the right eye together with blurring of vision and double vision suggests transient orbital ischaemia caused by reduced flow in the ophthalmic artery which arises from the internal carotid artery, and partial III nerve impairment resulting from ischaemia or compression of the oculomotor nerve which runs close to the internal carotid artery. Horner's syndrome occurs in association with dissection (see below and above case) but this causes a partial rather than complete ptosis and would not by itself cause diplopia.

Pulsatile tinnitus suggests carotid dissection but there are several alternative diagnoses that should have been considered in these cases. **Atheromatous carotid bifurcation stenosis** has been reported to be associated with a III nerve palsy but although bruits may be found on examination, pulsatile tinnitus would not be expected and would be unlikely to develop suddenly. **Carotid aneurysms** may cause tinnitus, bruits and oculomotor nerve abnormalities but would be unlikely to be bilateral in contrast to dissection, which often occurs in multiple vessels (see below). **Cavernous sinus thrombosis** can cause ocular pain and suffusion and abnormalities of the III, IV, VI, and V1 cranial nerves and lesions in the cavernous sinus may extend to the carotid artery leading to stroke (see page 132), and thus would be an alternative diagnosis in case B. However, cavernous sinus thrombosis usually causes pain and one would not expect relapsing and remitting symptoms. Finally, **carotico-cavernous fistulas** (and other vascular malformations (see Fig. 19.1)) may cause tinnitus together with a steal phenomenon resulting in ocular and cerebral ischaemia. These usually occur as a result of trauma, aneurysmal rupture, or underlying connective tissue disorder.

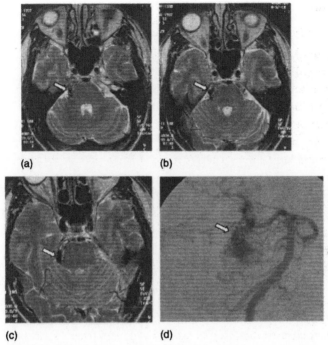

(a)　　　　　　　　　(b)

(c)　　　　　　　　　(d)

Fig. 19.1 T2-weighted MRI (a–c) and cerebral angiogram (d) showing a dural AV malformation (arrows) at the right cerebellopontine angle causing tinnitus.

19b) CT brain imaging is insensitive for detecting dissection although CT angiogram is becoming more widely available and may demonstrate stenosis and/or intramural haematoma. Carotid duplex may be suggestive of a dissection with high resistance flow in the distal internal carotid artery and absence of atheroma. However, axial MRI (from day 3) with MRA is usually necessary with images through the lesion showing a semilunar shaped haematoma in the arterial wall or absent flow void in affected vessels (see Figs. 19.2 and 19.3). Convential angiography (see Fig. 19.4) is indicated in those cases where non-invasive imaging is not diagnostic. Definite diagnosis may be required in trauma cases for legal purposes or insurance claims.

In case A, The T2-weighted MRI brain scan (Fig. 19.2) showed a right frontal infarct and lesions in the deep white matter on the right. On MRA, there was absence of a flow void in the right internal carotid artery and dissection of the left carotid with partial occlusion. Conventional angiography confirmed the MRA findings and showed that the vertebral arteries were probably normal.

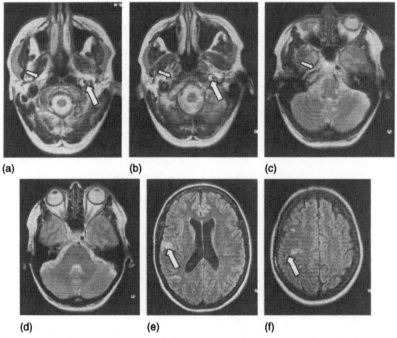

Fig. 19.2 MRI from case A showing bilateral carotid dissections with frontal infarction. A–d: The normal flow void is absent in the right carotid artery (small arrow) consistent with occlusion and there is partial occlusion of the left carotid artery (large arrow). C and F show an area of right frontal hyperintensity consistent with infarction (large arrows).

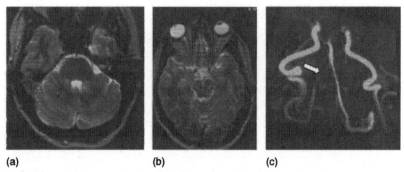

Fig. 19.3 Cerebellar and brain stem infarction on T2-weighted MRI (a, b) secondary to right vertebral dissection with occlusion of the right vertebral artery on MRA (arrow) (c).

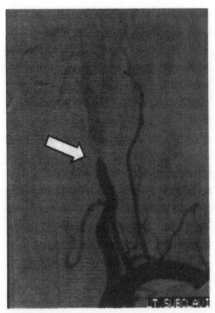

Fig. 19.4. Conventional angiogram showing focal left vertebral artery dissection (arrow) in a patient presenting with a history suggestive of SAH (see page 140).

In case B), the T2-weighted MRI brain scan showed a white dot in the region of the right carotid artery. MRA showed an occluded right internal carotid but no intramural thrombus was seen, meaning that occlusion on the background of atheromatous carotid stenosis could not be excluded. The left carotid artery was normal. Right carotid duplex confirmed vessel occlusion and no atheroma was seen.

19c) In arterial dissection, blood splits the wall of the vessel between the intima and the adventitia to form a false lumen.

The blood may enter via an intimal tear or may arise form vasavasorum rupture within the vessel wall. This may reduce the diameter of the true lumen, create a slow flowing false lumen, result in thrombus formation, and/or generate a dissecting aneurysm. Dissection may occur anywhere in the extracranial carotid artery. In the vertebral artery, the distal third is usually affected. Occasionally, aortic dissection may extend into the vertebral arteries and the carotids.

The incidence of diagnosed internal carotid dissection is around 1–4 per 100 000 per year. Vertebral dissection (see Figs. 19.3 and 19.4) is a little less common. The actual incidence of dissection is likely to be considerably higher, but the diagnosis is often missed, particularly in older patients.

Usually only one artery is involved but in about 10% of cases multiple arteries may be affected simultaneously or in close succession. Recurrence rates are low at around 1% per annum except in familial cases of arterial dissection or hereditary connective tissue disorder where rates are higher. Cranial artery dissection may result in stroke or TIA, retinal infarction or ischaemic oculopathy and spinal cord infarction (from vertebral and thus anterior spinal artery involvement) may occur without causing cerebral ischaemia. Although dissection may occur in association with connective tissue disease (see below), there is usually no known underlying abnormality. In one series, skin biopsy connective tissue abnormalities were reported in 68% of patients without clinical evidence of a hereditary connective tissue disorder supporting the hypothesis of a primary arteriopathy in these patients. There is also an unexplained association between dissection and migraine.

19d) Spontaneous dissection may occur in a variety of connective tissue diseases/syndromes including:

- Ehlers–Danlos
- Osler–Weber–Rendu
- Marfan
- Osteogenesis imperfecta
- Pseudoxanthoma elasticum
- Alpha1 antitrypsin deficiency
- Fibromuscular dysplasia
- Cystic medial necrosis.

Arterial dissection is also associated with syphilis.

19e) There are a number of diagnostic pointers to cervical arterial dissection which should be looked for in the history and examination:

- Possible neck injury including minor or major trauma (e.g. road traffic accident)
- Chiropractic manipulation
- Neck surgery
- Leaning back over hairdressers' sinks
- Labour
- Head banging
- Pain in the neck, side of the head, face or eye ipsilateral to the dissection in the case of the internal carotid artery and unilateral (usually) pain at the back of the head and neck for vertebral dissection.

- Horner's syndrome as a result of damage to sympathetic nerves around the internal carotid artery (occurring in up to 50%)

- Bruit audible to the patient which may be described as tinnitus owing to dissection adjacent to the base of the skull (occurring in about 30%)

- Ipsilateral palsy of a cranial nerve (12% in one series), often the XII or other lower cranial nerve, rarely the III nerve

- Cervical root lesions have been reported in association with vertebral artery dissections from pressure or ischaemia.

The presence of cranial neuropathy may result in a misdiagnosis of brainstem stroke. Cranial nerve palsies may result from local pressure from the false lumen or thromboembolism or haemodynamic compromise to the blood supply of the nerve. The III nerve receives its blood supply from the ophthalmic artery, branches of the internal carotid or the posterior cerebral artery and thus may become ischaemic after carotid dissection. However, this is very rare.

The features listed above may precede the onset of cerebral ischaemia by hours or days, and relevant points in the history may thus not be volunteered spontaneously by the patient. Alternatively, diagnostic pointers to dissection may be absent altogether and thus the diagnosis becomes one of exclusion/confirmation on imaging. Cervical arterial dissection generally has a benign prognosis (95% 10-year survival), although the risk of stroke is high during the first few days and weeks. Aneurysms do not appear to increase the risk of thromboembolism. However, massive MCA infarction may occur.

19f) There are no randomized controlled trials of treatment for cervical artery dissection, although anti-thrombotic treatment is generally advocated. It is unclear whether antiplatelet agents are superior to anticoagulants. Thrombolysis has been proposed in cases of complete thrombotic occlusion. Many physicians would treat acute recurrent ischaemic events with heparin.

Further reading

Mokri B, Silbert PL, Schievink WI, Piepgras DG (1996). Cranial nerve palsy in spontaneous dissection of the extracranial internal carotid artery. *Neurology*; 46(2):356–359.

Schievink WI (2001). Spontaneous dissection of the carotid and vertebral arteries. *N Engl J Med*; 344(12):898–906.

Case 20

A 42-year-old Spanish woman was brought to the emergency department with agitation, inappropriate behaviour, and vomiting. She had arrived in the UK a few days previously from Madrid. She had not been seen by her fellow students for 2 days and was found wandering naked, showing sexually inappropriate behaviour, and was agitated and uncooperative. She complained of diffuse abdominal pain and vomiting that had started 2 days previously. There was a past medical history of anorexia nervosa and depression. She denied taking any medication but laxatives were found in her pocket. On examination, she was thin, disorientated in time but orientated in place and person, agitated and restless, pacing around the cubicle. Her temperature was 36°C, pulse 120/min regular, and blood pressure 165/80mmHg. Examination was otherwise normal.

Initial investigations showed:

- Hb 16g/dL, WCC 15×10^9/L (84% neutrophils), platelets 232×10^9/L.
- CRP<8mg/L.
- Na 139mmol/L, K 3.7mmol/L, urea 7.5mmol/L, Cr 89µmol/L, Ca 2.44mmol/L, glucose 4.0mmol/L, AST 50IU/L, alk phos 330IU/L.
- ABG: pH 7.24, pO_2 14.2kPa, pCO_2 3.6kPa, base excess -14.8mmol/L, lactate 0.7mmol/L (0.6–1.2mmol/L), bicarbonate 12.3mmol/L, chloride 104mmol/L.

Questions

20a) Give a differential diagnosis.

20b) What do the blood gas results show?

20c) Give 3 causes of this type of blood gas abnormality.

20d) What is the most likely diagnosis taking into account the past medical history and the clinical findings?

20e) What are the neurological features of this condition?

20f) What further investigations would you perform in order to confirm your diagnosis?

20g) What is the treatment?

Answers

20a) The differential diagnosis is of an acute encephalopathy and is wide including:

- Acute psychosis/mania.
- Metabolic encephalopathy:
  - Hepatic/renal failure
  - Drugs
  - Electrolyte disturbance
  - Porphyria (see page 65).
- Endocrine disorder:
  - Hypoglycaemia
  - Hyperthyroidism
  - Hypercalcaemia.
- CNS infection.
- Space occupying lesion.
- Inflammatory disorders:
  - Demyelination
  - Vasculitis.
- CVT (see page 14)
- Head injury.
- Seizure:
  - Post ictal state
  - Non-convulsive status (see page 186).
- Catatonia.

20b) The blood gas results show a metabolic acidosis with normal lactate and an increased anion gap.

Metabolic acidosis may occur with a normal (bicarbonate loss or H+ ion ingestion) or increased (increased organic or inorganic acids) anion gap. The anion gap is calculated by the following formula: $(Na + K) - (Cl + HCO_3)$, giving a gap of $(139 + 3.7) - (104 + 2.3) = 26.4 mmol/L$ in this patient (normal range 10–18mmol/L).

20c) The causes of a metabolic acidosis with an increased anion gap are:

- Ketoacidosis:
  - Type I diabetes mellitus
  - Alcohol
  - Starvation.

- Drugs
  - Salicylates
  - Methanol
  - Ethylene glycol
  - Paraldehyde.
- Uraemia.
- Lactic acidosis:
  - Sepsis
  - Hypoxia.

20d) The diagnosis is **severe thyrotoxicosis (thyroid storm)** from thyrotoxicosis factitia (excess ingestion of thyroxine).

The abnormal investigations make it unlikely that a psychiatric disorder alone is responsible for this patient's symptoms. The elevated WCC and acidosis might initially suggest sepsis but the lactate and CRP were normal. A drug overdose is possible especially in view of the past medical history but a toxicology screen was negative. In this patient, the normal lactate, urea and glucose exclude the more common causes of metabolic acidosis with increased anion gap, leaving only starvation and alcohol. Ketonuria would be expected in both of these conditions.

Further inquiry revealed that the patient's uncle was a pharmacist. Investigation showed total T_4 227mmol/L (70–140mmol/L), free T_4 57.8mmol/L (9–25mmol/L), TSH<0.08mu/L, T_3 2.9mmol/L (1–2.5mmol/L) and decreased iodine uptake on radionucleotide scanning. Subacute thyroiditis would show reduced uptake on scanning but there was no neck pain, fever or raised inflammatory markers suggestive of this diagnosis. The relatively high T_4 to T_3 ratio is characteristic of exogenous excess thyroxine consumption as is the low thyroglobulin (present in thyroid follicles and released into the blood) level found in this patient (thyroglobulin undetectable at <5µg/L (normal <35µg/L)). Thyroglobulin is increased in endogenous hyperthyroidism. Further proof of thyrotoxicosis factitia can be obtained by demonstrating increased faecal thyroxine excretion and normal urinary iodine excretion to rule out exogenous excess iodine consumption.

20e) The neurological features of thyroid storm, often of abrupt onset, include:

- Confusion
- Agitation
- Restlessness

- Tremor
- Psychosis
- Hyperkinesis
- Chorea
- Encephalopathy
- Seizures.

Rarely coma, on a background of decreased mentation and apathy, may be seen particularly in the elderly, so-called 'apathetic hyperthyroidism'. Basal ganglia infarction and longterm cognitive impairment have been described. Myopathy and rhabdomyolysis may occur (see page 111). Non-neurological features include vomiting, abdominal pain, diarrhoea, fever, sweating, tachycardia/arrhythmia, heart failure, jaundice, and electrolyte derangement, many of which are illustrated by this case. Hepatic failure may be a present. Metabolic acidosis may occur but is usually caused by excess lactate.

20f) Untreated thyroid storm is fatal. This patient received Lugol's iodine to block endogenous thyroid hormone release, beta-blockers and carbimazole and dexamethasone to inhibit thyroid hormone release and block conversion of T4 to T3.

Further reading

Bogazzi F, Bartalena L, Scarcello G (1999). The age of patients with thyrotoxicosis factitia in Italy from 1973 to 1996. *J Endocrinol Invest*; 22(2):128–133.

Pearce CJ, Himsworth RL (1982). Thyrotoxicosis factitia. *N Engl J Med*; 307(27):1708–1709. No abstract available.

Sarlis NJ, Gourgiotis L (2003). Thyroid emergencies. *Rev Endocr Metab Disord*; 4(2):129–136

Case 21

A 22-year-old woman complained of having difficulty eating, and of closing her right eye. There was a history of otitis media 3 weeks previously for which she had received antibiotics. On examination, there was a complete right lower motor neuron VII palsy and she was given steroids and aciclovir for presumptive Bell's palsy. Over the next 4 days she developed bilateral hearing loss accompanied by severe right frontal and periorbital pain, worse on coughing. The following day she had double vision on looking to the right. Examination confirmed altered sensation over the V1 and V2 distribution, a right VI nerve palsy, right lower motor neuron VII and bilateral sensorineural hearing loss.

Questions

21a) What is the eponymous name of this syndrome?

21b) What are the neuroanatomical substrates of this syndrome?

21c) What are the most commonly associated organisms and what is the treatment?

21d) What other complications may occur with this condition?

21e) How would you investigate these patients radiologically?

Answers

21a) The diagnosis is **Gradenigo's syndrome**

In 1907, Giuseppe Gradenigo described a syndrome of otitis media, facial pain (pain in the division of V1 and V2), and an ipsilateral VI nerve palsy [the first case with added VII and VIII nerve palsies (see below)]. It is caused by infection from the middle ear spreading to the petrous temporal bone ('petrous apicitis'). This was a common complication of middle ear infection in the pre–antibiotic era. Petrous apicitis may not be associated with the complete triad of symptoms described by Gradenigo, or alternatively there may be other cranial nerve deficits. Gradenigo's syndrome may also be used to describe a similar pattern of neurological deficits caused by pathological processes affecting the petrous temporal bone other than extension of infection from otitis media.

21b) The petrous apex is a pyramidal shaped bone lying between the inner ear and the clivus in the most medial portion of the temporal bone. In 30% of individuals, the petrous temporal bone contains air cells that communicate with the middle-ear cleft providing a route for spread of infection from the middle ear. Infection may be acute with abscess formation and rapidly progressive symptoms or chronic and associated with osteomyelitis.

The V (trigeminal ganglion) and VI nerves are the two most commonly affected cranial nerves in petrous apicitis since they are separated from the petrous bone only by a thin layer of dura mater. Deficits in other cranial nerves, II–XII can occur depending on whether the infectious process extends to the skull base or cavernous sinus. Direct extension of infection may involve the VIII nerve and lead to vertigo and hearing loss. Facial nerve paralysis may occur as seen in the first case above and Bell's palsy should be diagnosed with caution in patients with associated otitis media in case petrous apicitis is overlooked.

21c) Early recognition and treatment of Gradenigo's syndrome is important to prevent complications, many of which are life-threatening (see below). The most commonly associated infectious agents are *Staphylococcus aureus* and *Pseudomonas aeruginosa*. Streptococcus, haemophilus, and TB have also been reported. Initial antibiotic therapy should thus be broad and antibiotics should be continued for at least 2–3 weeks and for 6 weeks where there is associated osteomyelitis. Abscess formation requires surgery.

21d) Complications of Gradenigo's syndrome include:

- Meningitis
- CVT (otic hydrocephalus) (see page 14).
- Mastoiditis
- Subdural empyema (see page 259)
- Cerebritis
- Cerebral abscess.

21e) CT scan of the sinuses and temporal bones is the initial investigation of choice.

CT shows inflammatory change in the petrous temporal bone (opacification or coalescence of the petrous air cells). Subperiosteal lucency indicates possible abscess formation, the latter will enhance with contrast. Destruction of bone resembling osteomyelitis indicates chronic apicitis. There may be associated opacification of the ipsilateral mastoid cells. MRI may be performed to provide better soft tissue visualization (see Fig. 21.1).

Further reading

Sherman SC and Buchanan A (2004). Gradenigo syndrome: A case report and review of a rare complication of otitis media. *J Emerg Med;* **27**:253–256.

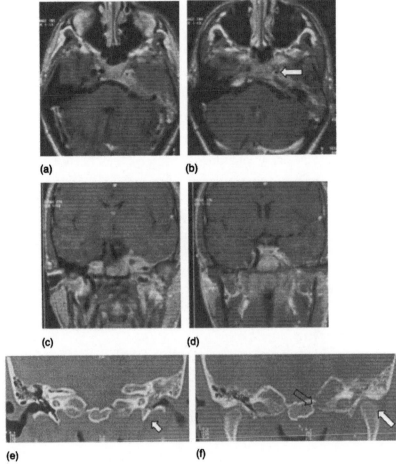

Fig. 21.1 MRI brain axial (a,b) and coronal T1 weighted contrast enhanced (c,d) scan shows pathological enhancement of the left petrous apex, Meckel's cave and cavernous sinus. The left carotid artery (arrow) runs through the inflammatory mass and is narrowed by it. The inflammatory tissue in the petrous apex is contiguous with material in the middle air cleft and mastoid. Coronal CT scans of the petrous bone (e,f) show a completely normal right ear but extensive opacity of the middle ear cleft (small arrow) and mastoid (large arrow) on the left. The left petrous apex shows some early bony erosion (open arrow).

Case 22

A 25-year-old man presented with a left hemiparesis. There was a two-week history of right jaw and posterior neck pain, headache, fevers, cough, anorexia, and weight loss. A few days prior to onset of these symptoms he had had a sore throat. He had a past history of otits media, but had otherwise been healthy.

On examination he was pyrexial at 39°C and agitated with a GCS of 14. There was tender cervical lymphadenopathy and a painful stiff neck (worse on the right) and he was holding his head to the right. The right eye was proptosed with injected conjunctivae. Neurological examination showed normal fundi, a right Horner's syndrome, a left homonymous hemianopia, right VI nerve palsy and left upper motor neuron VII. There was a left hemiparesis.

Investigations showed:

- Hb 12.6g/dL, WCC 26 × 10⁹/L (23 × 10⁹/L neutrophils), platelets 363 × 10⁹/L, CRP 160mg/L, Na 128mmol/L, LFT normal
- CXR: bilateral focal lesions and left pleural effusion
- CT brain: unremarkable
- CSF: glucose <1mmol/L (blood 5mmol/L), protein 1.8g/dL, red cells 50/mm³, polymorphs 1000/mm³
- MRI/MRA brain is shown in Fig. 22.1.

Questions

22a) What abnormalities are indicated by the arrows on the MRI/MRA?

22b) What is the eponymous name given to the condition illustrated by this case?

22c) What complications have occurred in this case?

22d) Which organism is likely to be responsible? What is the treatment?

22e) With which other clinical syndromes is this organism associated?

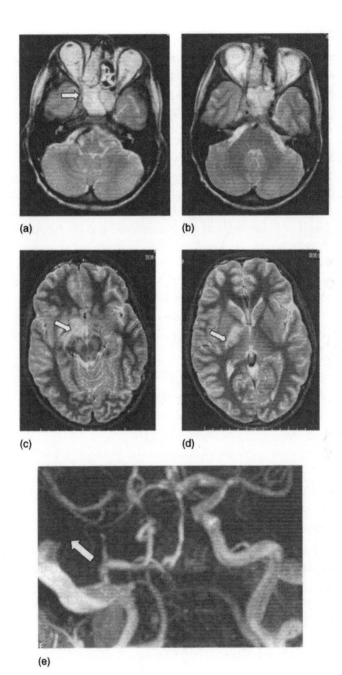

Fig. 22.1

Answers

22a) The T2–weighted MRI (Fig. 22.1) shows opacification of the sphenoid sinuses (a and b) and deep right hemisphere infarction (c and d). The MRA shows a tight right carotid stenosis/occlusion (e).

22b) The eponymous name given to this condition is **Lemierre's syndrome**.

This patient has the clinical features of Lemierre's syndrome (Lemierre's postanginal septicaemia), which often affects previously healthy young adults. There is a male preponderance. It is characterized by a sore throat followed by painful cervical lymphadenopathy, systemic upset and spread of infection to the parapharyngeal tissue causing pain and induration at the angle of the jaw, internal jugular vein thrombosis, and septicaemia. Metastatic spread of infection characteristically affects the lungs causing septic infarcts but may also involve bone, joint, liver, brain, and heart valves. CXR may show cavitating or nodular lesions, pneumothorax, effusion, empyema or abscess. Evidence of the primary oropharyngeal infection may have vanished by the time the patient presents, and misdiagnosis as infectious endocarditis is not uncommon.

22c) The complications that have occurred in this patient are:

- Cavernous sinus thrombophlebitis
- Right carotid artery thromboembolism causing left cerebral ischaemia
- Right internal jugular thrombophlebitis
- Meningitis.

Cavernous sinus thrombosis/thrombophlebitis is frequently associated with sepsis of head and neck structures and should be considered in patients who develop any combination of unilateral chemosis, proptosis and diplopia with variable involvement of cranial nerves II, III, IV, V1, V2, and VI. The symptoms and signs are usually unilateral initially but often progress to involve the other eye because the venous plexus communicates across the midline. Thrombosis may also extend into the other venous sinuses. The left-sided homonymous hemianopia and left hemiparesis seen in this patient indicate a right hemisphere lesion. Right carotid artery thromboembolism with associated Horner's syndrome is the likely mechanism since the internal carotid artery passes through the cavernous sinus. The right neck pain is likely to be secondary to right internal jugular thrombophlebitis from direct spread of infection or from venous drainage from the cavernous sinus.

The CSF neutrophil leukocytosis, low glucose and elevated protein indicate an associated bacterial meningitis.

Alternative diagnoses in this patient include i) infective endocarditis (see page 148) with mycotic aneurysms causing infarcts in the right pons and the right cerebral cortex and secondary cavernous sinus thrombosis and ii) meningitis with associated cerebral venous sinus thrombosis, but neither of these explain the temporal sequence of symptoms nor all the clinical features seen in this patient.

22d) The organism responsible for Lemierre's syndrome is *Fusobacterium necrophorum*, an anaerobic organism that is normally present in the oropharynx.

Necrobacillosis is the term given to septicaemia caused by this organism with postanginal septicaemia designated as Lemierre's disease as this is a distinct entity. Urgent CT/MRI is indicated. The airway should be monitored closely as obstruction may occur. Patients require prolonged antibiotic treatment with penicillin and metronidazole or clindamycin and drainage of collections. Antithrombotic treatments are often advocated. Prior to antibiotics, the mortality from the condition was around 80%. Although mortality is now much reduced, significant morbidity remains.

22e) In addition to throat infection, *Fusobacterium necrophorum* causes infection of the skin and subcutaneous tissues (necrotising fasciitis), otitis media and mastoiditis, genital, alimentary and urinary tract infection and empyema.

Further reading

Lemierre A (1936). On certain septicaemias due to anaerobic organisms. *Lancet*; 1:701–703.

Moreno S, Garcia Altozano J, Pinilla B, *et al.* (1989). Lemierre's disease: postanginal bacteremia and pulmonary involvement caused by Fusobacterium necrophorum. *Rev Infect Dis*; 11(2):319–324.

Plymyer MR, Zoccola DG, Tallarita G (2004). Pathologic quiz case: an 18-year-old man presenting with sepsis following a recent pharyngeal infection. Lemierre syndrome. *Arch Pathol Lab Med*; 128(7):813–814

Case 23

An 80-year-old man was admitted to hospital having been found drowsy and slumped to the left in a chair by a neighbour. He had been well until 3 weeks prior to admission when he had developed a cough productive of green sputum. His GP had treated him for a presumptive chest infection with a course of amoxycillin. However, he failed to improve and became more short of breath, whereupon he was prescribed clarithromycin and frusemide. On the day of admission he had become progressively more drowsy. There was a past history of hypertension and he had had a stroke 6 years previously, from which he had made a complete recovery. He lived alone and was usually independent and self-caring. Medications were aspirin, bendrofluazide, furosemide, and doxazosin.

On examination, the temperature was 36°C, pulse was 110/min regular, BP was 150/80 mmHg, and BM was 6.8mmol/L. He was mildly dehydrated, the jugular venous pressure was not elevated and the cardiac apex was displaced with a quiet systolic murmur. There was no oedema. There were coarse crepitations at the right lung base and oxygen saturation was 95% on air. He was drowsy with a fluctuating GCS of 13–15 and was disorientated in time but not in place or person. There was no evidence of cranial nerve deficit except that his swallow was felt to be unsafe. Tone was normal in all limbs, but he had moderate weakness in the left arm and leg and an upgoing left plantar. The right limbs were normal.

Investigations showed:

- Hb 11.3g/dL, WCC 8.8 × 10⁹/L, plat 258 × 10⁹/L
- Na 111mmol/L, K 3.7mmol/L, urea 7mmol/L, Cr 76μmol/L, Ca 2.24mmol/L, PO$_4$ 1.04mmol/L, alb 34g/L
- CRP 137mg/L
- CXR: cardiomegaly, unfolded calcified aorta, small pleural effusions, minor right basal consolidation
- ECG: normal axis, sinus rhythm, lateral T-wave flattening.

Cerebral imaging was performed and treatment was started. By the next day, he was much improved with no evidence of neurological deficit.

Questions

23a) What are the 3 most likely causes of this man's focal neurological signs?

23b) What is the likely sequence of events leading to his admission?

23c) What treatment would you have given?

23d) Why are elderly patients more prone to develop hyponatraemia?

Answers

23a) The 3 most likely causes of this man's focal neurological signs are:

- Hyponatraemia causing focal deficit directly or via a seizure with a residual hemiparesis
- Stroke
- Cerebral abscess.

The sodium was very low at 111 (see page 182 for further discussion of the neurological manifestations of hyponatraemia). Focal neurological signs may be seen in the setting of **hyponatraemia** and include hemiparesis, monoparesis, ataxia, tremor, nystagmus, dysphasia, and unilateral corticospinal tract signs. There is often, but not always, an underlying structural lesion. The signs resolve with correction of the sodium abnormality. The rapid resolution of his symptoms, together with the rise in Na to 132mmol/L one day following admission, suggest that this was the most likely cause of his symptoms.

Hyponatraemia also causes seizures. It is possible that this patient may have had an unwitnessed seizure followed by a residual **(Todd's) hemiparesis**. The previous history of chest infection followed by drowsiness and focal neurological abnormality raises the possibility of **cerebral abscess**.

This patient has a past history of cerebrovascular disease, hypertension and has cardiomegaly, making him at high risk of **recurrent stroke**. It is therefore possible that he has had a further cerebrovascular event. This was not shown on the CT scan but since the sensitivity of CT for ischaemic stroke is limited, a further ischaemic event cannot be excluded. Diffusion weighted MRI would be of diagnostic value (see page 31) as it has high sensitivity for recent stroke, allowing distinction to be made between old and acute stroke.

23b) This patient developed a respiratory tract infection in the community and received appropriate treatment. However, his symptoms failed to improve and he was given diuretics. The combination of chest infection causing increased ADH secretion together with increased renal sodium loss from thiazide and loop diuretics is the likely cause of his low sodium.

23c) Treatment includes:

- Intravenous antibiotics
- Cessation of diuretics
- Rehydration with normal saline.

Intravenous antibiotics were given for community acquired pneumonia. He was not felt to be in left ventricular failure at the time of admission. The frusemide and bendrofluazide were stopped. He was kept nil by mouth initially owing to his poor swallow and received 2L of normal saline over 24 hours to maintain his hydration. The rise in sodium was perhaps faster than that recommended (see page 183) but he suffered no ill effects. It is likely that the hyponatraemia had developed subacutely in line with his respiratory illness and there is evidence that rapid correction of hyponatraemia is less likely to cause complications when the decline in sodium has occurred rapidly than when hyponatraemia has become chronic (see page 183).

The correct treatment of hyponatraemia depends on accurate assessment of the patient's hydration status, which in turn determines the likely cause of the hyponatraemia. Urine and plasma osmolarity and urinary sodium concentration are helpful but can only be interpreted in the light of hydration status. Hypovolaemic hyponatraemia occurs in association with vomiting and diarrhoea, overdiuresis, renal tubular salt wasting, and mineralocorticoid deficiency. These patients should be treated by replacement of water and sodium loss (usually with normal saline) together with cessation of any implicated drugs. Euvolaemic hyponatraemia occurs commonly in elderly patients who are unwell for other reasons and who are taking diuretics but is also seen in SIADH (an overdiagnosed condition). These patients respond to fluid restriction and treatment of underlying conditions and cessation of medication where applicable. Hypervolaemic hyponatraemia occurs in cardiac, liver and renal failure in which there is an excess of both sodium and water. These patients should receive water and sodium restriction together with treatment of the underlying disorder.

23c) Elderly patients are more prone to develop hyponatraemia because of:

- Increased ADH secretion for a given osmolality
- Medication
- Presence of concomitant illness.

Hyponatraemia is the most common electrolyte abnormality found in hospitalized patients and is particularly found in elderly people in whom it is usually multifactorial. The neurological consequences of low plasma sodium are a frequent cause of admission of elderly patients to hospital. Elderly patients are often on medications causing water retention or renal sodium loss and are more likely to respond adversely to factors causing haemodilution. There is a small decline in renal concentrating ability with age, but the renal response to exogenous ADH appears to be unrelated to age. Older people tend to have higher ADH secretions for a given osmolality and hormone measuremements show increased hypothalamic ADH content with age. Further, elderly people show greater rises in ADH secretion with hypertonic saline. Taken together, this suggests augmented ADH secretion with age in the absence of reduced renal sensitivity. This may explain why elderly people are more likely to become hyponatraemic in the face of physiological stressors or medication.

Further reading

Huff JS (2002). Stroke mimics and chameleons. *Emerg Med Clin North Am;* **20**(3):583–585.

Case 24

Two cases are presented below.

Case A A 53-year-old woman presented to the emergency department with a sudden onset severe occipital headache that had developed at rest. There was no associated vomiting or loss of consciousness. There was no past history of migraine or other headache. She was married and working as a business analyst. On examination, she was alert and orientated, fundi were normal and there was no neck stiffness or neurological abnormality.

Case B A 39-year-old male policeman presented to the emergency department with sudden onset generalized headache that had occurred whilst he was sitting watching television. There were no associated symptoms apart from mild confusion. On examination, his GCS was 14 and he was disorientated in place and time.

In case A, CT brain was unremarkable but subsequent LP showed xanthochromia. In case B, the CT showed SAH. Both patients went on to have cerebral angiograms that did not demonstrate any aneurysm.

Questions

24a) What are the time intervals for which brain CT and CSF xanthochromia may be positive after SAH? If SAH had been excluded in these two cases, what other two important alternative diagnoses should have been considered?

24b) What specific pattern of bleeding on CT is particularly associated with angiogram negative SAH?

24c) Give 5 possible causes of angiogram negative SAH.

24d) Would you investigate these patients further?

Answers

24a) Any case of suspected SAH requires an urgent CT brain and if this is negative an LP should be performed to look for xanthochromia.

CT will demonstrate blood in more than 95% of patients in the first 48 hours after onset but this falls rapidly to 50% on day 7 and almost nil at day 10. Moreover, CT evidence is sometimes subtle and easily missed without expert neuroradiological input. LP should be performed at least 12 hours after onset to allow red cell break down to produce oxyhaemoglobin and bilirubin. Xanthochromia may be detectable in the CSF up to 4 weeks after onset but a normal CSF examination after 2 weeks does not exclude SAH. Patients who have a positive CT or LP should have a cerebral angiogram to look for aneurysms. SAH is caused by a ruptured aneurysm in 85% of cases, nonaneurysmal perimesencephalic bleeding in 10% (see below) and various rare conditions in 5%. Case fatality is around 50% and one-third remain dependent. If SAH is excluded and the patient remains unwell, alternative diagnoses should be considered including cerebral venous sinus thrombosis and occult CNS infection.

24b) **Perimesencephalic blood only** (blood confined to the cisterns around the midbrain) since perimesencephalic SAH is the most common cause of angiogram negative SAH (see below).

24c) The causes of angiogram negative SAH include:

- False negative angiogram
- Perimesencephalic SAH
- Occult vascular malformation
- Arterial dissection
- Head trauma
- Vasculitis
- Other (see below).

In up to 20% of CT or LP positive SAH (a traumatic LP may be misdiagnosed as xanthochromic) the cerebral angiogram shows no aneurysm, so called '**angiogram negative SAH**'. Angiogram negative SAH results when there is a **false negative angiogram (2–23%)** or when the SAH was caused by something other than an intracerebral aneurysm. The pattern of subarachnoid bleeding is an important clue as to whether the bleed is likely to have been caused by an underlying aneurysm. Patients with diffuse or anteriorly located blood (an aneurysmal pattern of haemorrhage) on CT (see Fig. 24.1) are at risk of rebleeding and repeat angiography should be performed in such cases as well as in cases where the previous angiogram was inadequate, or views were incomplete owing to vasospasm or haemorrhage.

In two thirds of patients with angiogram negative SAH, the CT shows **perimesencephalic blood** (see Fig. 24.2). Patients with perimesencephalic SAH present, usually in their sixth decade, with acute onset headache. Loss of consciousness, focal symptoms and seizures are rare. The cause of perimesencephalic SAH is usually unknown but it has an invariably good prognosis since rebleeding and vasospasm are extremely unlikely. Aneurysms of the basilar and vertebral arteries may occasionally (2.5–5% of perimesencephalic SAH) cause extravasation of blood into the midbrain cisterns. Many physicians perform CT angiography rather than catheter angiography in patients with perimesencephalic SAH as the risks of catheter angiography are felt to outway the small risk of not diagnosing a posterior circulation aneurysm with CT angiography.

Causes of SAH in which the angiogram is truly negative, besides perimesencephalic SAH, include **occult vascular malformation, arterial dissection** (almost always in the posterior circulation) (see page 117), **head trauma, cardiac myxoma, coagulopathy, sickle cell anaemia, vasculitis** (see page 175), **CVT** (see page 14), **drugs (e.g. amphetamine and cocaine), pituitary apoplexy** (see page 300), **sickle cell anaemia, mycotic aneurysm** (see page 150) and spinal abnormalities such as **dural and cord arterio-venous malformation** (see page 280) **or cavernous angioma**. In cases where the cause of SAH remains unclear, the history and examination should be reviewed along with the radiology. MRI should be considered as this may demonstrate an arteriovenous malformation or tumour. Spine radiology should be considered especially if blood is seen in the foramen magnum or other features suggest a spinal problem.

24d) Repeat cerebral angiography if the first study is inadequate. Consider further imaging including MRI/angiography of the cervical spine especially if blood is seen in the foramen magnum.

In case A, a cervical angiogram showed a C1/C2 dural arterio-venous fistula which was treated surgically with cervical laminectomy and division of the fistula. In case B, an arteriovenous fistula at the base of the brain was found (see Fig. 24.3).

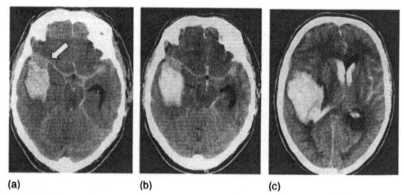

(a)   (b)   (c)

Fig. 24.1 CT scan from a patient with rupture of an aneursym (arrow) showing aneurysmal haemorrhage pattern with blood extending into the subarachnoid space and into the right hemisphere forming a haematoma rupturing into the ventricular system. There is midline shift with ventricular distortion.

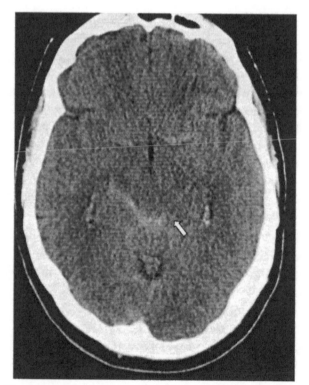

Fig. 24.2 CT scan showing perimesencephalic SAH with blood in the basal cisterns only (arrow).

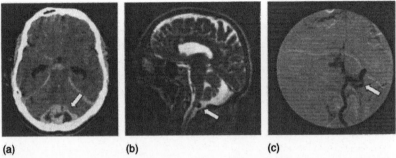

Fig. 24.3 Neuroimaging from case B): CT (a) showing dilute blood in the prepontine system and blood in the cisternal magna (arrow) which has clotted and retracted. T2-weighted MRI (b) shows a prominent collection of vessels around the medulla (arrow). The AP vertebral angiogram (c) shows no onward flow into the basilar artery and early drainage of veins into the epidural venous plexus (arrow) indicating an arteriovenous fistula.

Further reading

Rinkel JE, van Gijn J, Wijdicks EFM (1993). Subarachnoid hemorrhage without detectable aneurysm: a review of the causes. *Stroke;* 23:1403–1409.

Van Gijn J and Rinkel GJE (2001). Subarachnoid haemorrhage: diagnosis, causes and management. *Brain;* 124:249–278.

Case 25

An 18-year-old woman was admitted overnight with a 2-day history of malaise, fever, and palpitations. There was no past medical history and she was taking no medication. She was unemployed and lived with her boyfriend. She smoked 20 cigarettes a day, and drank approximately 20 units of alcohol per week. She admitted to occasional use of heroin and cocaine.

On examination, she was febrile at 38°C with a tachycardia of 250/min regular and a blood pressure of 130/80 mmHg. There were needle track marks on her arms and vascular access was very difficult. She was warm and well perfused. Heart sounds were difficult owing to the tachycardia respiratory and abdominal examinations were unremarkable. There was a maculopapular rash over the feet and hands and swelling of the small joints of the hands. She was alert and orientated with no neck stiffness or photophobia and no focal neurological abnormality.

She was admitted and initial treatment including amiodarone was commenced. Her pulse rate dropped to 100/min.

Investigations showed:

- Hb 15.2g/dL, WCC 17.5 × 10⁹/L (88% neutrophils with toxic granulation), plt 48 × 10⁹/L
- PT 12.6 sec (10–13.5 sec), APTT 31.3 sec (22–34 sec)
- Na 126mmol/L, K 3.4mmol/L, urea 15.2mmol/L, Cr 131µmol/L, CRP 200mg/L, troponin 2.4mmol/L (mildly elevated), ALT 85IU/L, glc 7.7mmol/L, alb 31g/L, bilirubin 17mmol/L, alk phos 315IU/L
- CXR: normal heart size, lungs clear
- ECG: supraventricular arrythmia
- Urine dipstick: +++ blood, trace protein, no leucocytes or nitrite.

The following morning, she became suddenly more unwell, with drowsiness and inability to move her right side. She remained pyrexial with a pulse of 110/min regular and a blood pressure of 120/80mm Hg. The respiratory rate was raised at 40/min with oxygen saturations of 92% on air and a productive cough. Her GCS was 13, there was no response to visual threat from the right and reduced tone and severely reduced power on the right. The right plantar was upgoing. There was no evidence of dysphasia.

Questions

25a) What is the most likely underlying diagnosis?

25b) What are the criteria for establishing this diagnosis?

25c) What are the two most likely causes of her neurological deterioration, one of which is shown on this patient's CT brain in Fig. 25.1?

25d) What other neurological abnormalities may occur in association with this diagnosis?

25e) What other investigations would you request and what might you expect to find?

25f) Describe your management plan. Would you have anticoagulated this patient?

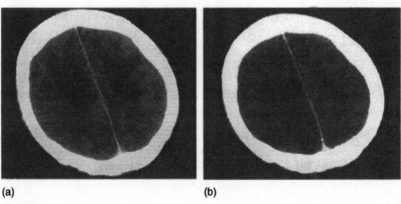

(a)   (b)

Fig. 25.1

Answers

25a) The most likely diagnosis is **infective endocarditis** caused by intravenous drug use.

Infective endocarditis is an important cause of stroke that should be considered especially in young patients without other obvious cause for stroke. This patient with fever is a known intravenous drug user and therefore at high risk of staphylococcal infections, including endocarditis. The presence of a cardiac arrhythmia in the absence of

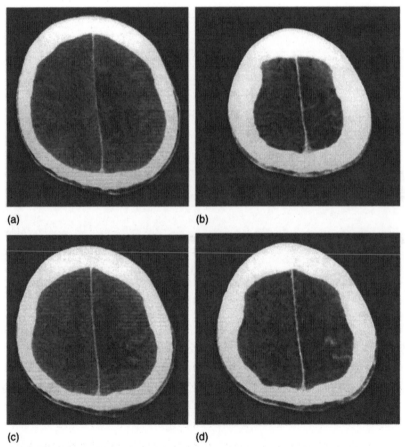

(a)   (b)

(c)   (d)

Fig. 25.2 CT brain (upper images without and lower images with contrast respectively) taken 1 week after onset of stroke showing hypodensity in the medial left hemisphere superiorly within the territory of the pericallosal artery. Areas of luxury perfusion are shown on the contrast enhanced images.

previous cardiac history, evidence of emboli to the peripheries and probably to the kidneys (haematuria) and brain strongly suggest this diagnosis (see below for diagnostic criteria). The triad of fever, heart murmur and hemiplegia was first described by Osler in the 1800s.

25b) The diagnosis of infectious endocarditis is based on the following criteria:

Major criteria

1) Two positive blood cultures with typical organism e.g. *S. viridans, S. bovis, S. aureus.*

2) Persistently positive blood cultures with other micro-organism consistent with endocarditis.

3) Evidence of endocardial involvement: positive echocardiogram for endocarditis and/or new valvular regurgitation.

Minor criteria

1) Predisposition: prior heart condition or intravenous drug abuse.

2) Fever >38°C.

3) Vascular phenomena e.g. emboli, septic pulmonary infarcts, intracranial haemorrhage, mycotic aneurysm, Janeway lesions.

4) Evidence of immune complex deposition e.g. Roth spots, purpuric rash, glomerulonephritis.

5) Microbiological evidence: positive blood culture not meeting major criteria or serological evidence of infection consistent with endocarditis.

6) Echocardiographic changes not meeting major criteria.

The diagnosis is considered definite if there are 2 major criteria, or 1 major and 3 minor, or 5 minor criteria.

This patient met all the major criteria and all the minor criteria not covered by the major criteria. Nine out of 10 (5 pairs) blood cultures were positive for methicillin sensitive *Staphylococcal aureus* (MRSA). There was evidence of renal infarction, hepatic infarction, splenic infarction and splenomegaly (see below).

25c) Possible causes of this patient's neurological deterioration are:

- Cerebral infarction caused by embolism from the heart, most likely from a vegetation on the mitral valve.

- Cerebral haemorrhage caused by pyogenic necrosis of the arterial wall or rupture of mycotic aneurysm (less likely).

The CT brain shows patchy hypodensity in the left parietal region consistent with ischaemic stroke. The CT abnormalities were more clearly seen on a subsequent scan taken a week later (see Fig. 25.2). Around one-fifth of patients with infective endocarditis have an ischaemic stroke as a result of embolism from valvular vegetations and the risk is thought to be higher with more virulent organisms. The cortex is usually involved consistent with an embolic aetiology. Cerebrovascular symptoms may be the presenting feature (around 20% of those with ischaemic stroke) but they usually occur in patients already hospitalized in whom infection is not already controlled. Haemorrhagic transformation is fairly common (18–42%). Cerebral emboli are probably not more common than emboli to other organs but are more frequently reported as they are usually symptomatic and associated with increased morbidity and mortality. Occasionally, emboli to the anterior spinal artery may cause paraplegia (see page 192).

Infective endocarditis is complicated by intracerebral haemorrhage in around 5% of cases. More than 80% of patients with intracerebral haemorrhage from septic emboli have a history of heart disease or intravenous drug abuse or prodromal symptoms suggestive of cerebral ischaemia. Cerebral haemorrhage in infective endocarditis is most commonly caused by pyogenic necrosis of the arterial wall early on in the disease, usually with virulent organisms such as *Staphylococcus aureus* and before effective treatment with antibiotics. Bleeding from ruptured mycotic aneurysms is less common but may occur later during antimicrobial therapy or with less virulent bacteria such as *Streptococcus viridans* or *Staphylococcus epidermidis*. Mycotic aneurysms most often affect the distal branches of the middle cerebral artery. They tend to resolve with time and thus angiography to detect aneurysms with a view to surgery is generally not warranted although some argue that it should be preformed in those with haemorrhagic stroke or in whom long term anticoagulation is being considered.

Given that fever, cardiac murmur and abnormal echocardiography are not always present in endocarditis, the diagnosis should always be considered in any patient with otherwise unexplained ischaemic or haemorrhagic stroke, particularly if there are elevated inflammatory markers, anaemia, persistent neutrophil leukocytosis, haematuria or disturbed liver function.

25d) Other neurological manifestations of infective endocarditis besides stroke include:

- Meningitis, cerebritis
- Encephalopathy
- Cerebral abscess/empyema (see page 258)
- Acute mononeuropathy
- Discitis (see page 168).

The frequency of neurological complications in infective endocarditis is in the region of 20–40%, of which ischaemic stroke is the most common, but the incidence varies with the infecting organism. Most neurological complications are caused by embolization and primary infection of the CNS without prior evidence of stroke is uncommon. Unsurprisingly, systemic embolic complications are more common with left sided cardiac involvement. Embolism from the right heart (which is more frequently involved in intravenous drug abusers than in other patients) is associated with patent foramen ovale or pulmonary arteriovenous malformation. Meningitis and cerebritis follow embolization to the meninges whereas embolization to the brain can cause micro- and macro-abscesses. Macro-abcesses are rare (fewer than 1% of neurological complications) and may occur within an area of infarction. Micro-abscesses are more common and may cause encephalopathy or psychosis. Embolization to the spinal meninges may cause a discitis and to the peripheral nerves may cause an ischaemic neuropathy in which persistent deep burning pain is the most common manifestation.

25e) Other investigations that should be requested in this patient include:

- Blood cultures: at least 3 sets taken at least 1 hour apart, ideally from different sites prior to starting antibiotics
- Echocardiography (transthoracic and transoesophageal)
- CT chest/CTPA and abdomen.

Echocardiography is mandatory to identify valvular vegetations and to assess cardiac function. Transthoracic echocardiography may be negative particularly with left sided lesions and trans-oesophageal echocardiography is nearly always required. In this patient (see Fig. 25.3), transthoracic echocardiography performed on the night of her admission, in which good views of the valves were seen, showed no evidence of abnormality. The following morning, however, repeat transthoracic studies showed thickening of the mitral valve with a small vegetation,

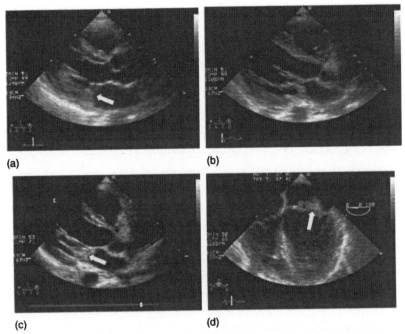

(a) (b) (c) (d)

Fig. 25.3 Echocardiogram images showing rapid progression of a lesion affecting the posterior leaflet of the mitral valve over a 32-hour period. a), b) and c) show parasternal long axis views from trans-thoracic echocardiography with an initially normal appearing posterior leaflet (a) with an increasingly thickened appearance from b) to c). d) is a four chamber view from a trans-oesophageal echocardiogram showing a large vegetation on the posterior mitral valve leaflet (arrow).

and trans-oesophageal echocardiography performed a few hours later showed a large mitral valve vegetation. There was no abnormality seen in the right heart. Rapid progression of symptoms and signs is common in patients with staphylococcal endocarditis and occurred in this patient despite institution of the correct antibiotic regimen at the time of her admission.

Although intravenous drug users are at higher risk of right heart endocarditis than other patients with endocarditis, the left heart is still more commonly affected owing to the higher pressures and greater turbulence of flow. In right heart endocarditis, septic pulmonary infarction may occur and was thought initially to be a possible cause of this patient's respiratory deterioration.

CT chest and abdomen was performed owing to the decline in respiratory function and haematuria. This showed right basal consolidation

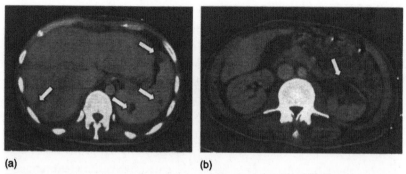

(a)   (b)

Fig. 25.4 CT abdomen from this patient showing hepatic, multiple splenic and left renal infarcts (arrows).

thought to be secondary to aspiration pneumonia, splenomegaly with splenic infarction and left renal infarction (see Fig. 25.4). There was no evidence of pulmonary infarction.

25f) Management of this patient includes:

- Prompt initiation of appropriate antibiotic therapy
- Liaison with microbiologist, cardiologist, and cardiothoracic surgeon
- Consideration of cardiac surgery
- Anticoagulation should not be given.

Prompt treatment with appropriate antibiotics is of paramount importance in the management of infective endocarditis since this reduces the risk of complications, particularly cerebral embolism. Numerous studies have shown a sharp reduction in the risk of embolism over the first few days of appropriate antibiotic therapy. Identification of the causative organism is required in guiding appropriate treatment and multiple sets of blood cultures should be taken. In a patient who is known to use intravenous drugs, *Staphylococcus aureus* would be the most likely causative organism. It should be noted that methicillin resistant strains are becoming more common in the community and intravenous drug users are at increased risk. Candida is also an important cause of endocarditis in drug users. Serological tests should be taken for Coxiella and Chlamydia in patients with negative blood cultures in whom the suspicion of endocarditis remains high.

Correct management of endocarditis requires close liaison between physicians, cardiologists, microbiologists, and cardiothoracic surgeons;

the latter should be notified even in the case of apparently stable patients, as rapid deterioration may occur. Early institution of the correct antibiotic regimen should be guided by microbiology advice. The indications for surgery are disputed but valvular deterioration, infection with resistant or virulent organisms or evidence of embolization have all been proposed. The presence of vegetations has not been shown consistently to be related to embolization although this is used as a criteria for surgery by some. The timing of surgery in patients with stroke is also controversial since the risks of early surgery in the presence of cerebral oedema have to be weighed against the risks of valvular deterioration or further embolization if surgery is delayed. This patient received a mitral valve replacement 36 hours after admission.

Early institution of the correct antibiotic therapy is the most effective way to prevent thromboembolism, the risks of which are highest in the first 24 – 48 hours after diagnosis. Anticoagulation should not be given to patients with native valve or bioprosthetic valve endocarditis because of the risk of intracerebral haemorrhage from mycotic aneurysms and arteritis and the reduction in embolism risk with antibiotic therapy. For patients with mechanical valves who are on long-term anticoagulation at the time of developing infective endocarditis, the correct management is unclear. Some advocate withholding anticoagulation in all such patients because it has not been shown to be associated with a reduction in the rate of systemic embolization and the risk of haemorrhagic complications with such therapy has been shown to be in the region of 40% in some studies. Others continue anticoagulation unless embolic stroke or haemorrhage occur. The length of time for which anticoagulation should be withheld is also unclear but consultation with the cardiologists regarding the risk of embolization according to valve type may be of some help. Some authors have stated that large ischaemic stroke, haemorrhage on CT, presence of mycotic aneurysm, uncontrolled infection and infection with *Staphylococcus aureus* are all contraindications to anticoagulants in mechanical valve endocarditis. There is no evidence for antiplatelet therapy in ischaemic stroke secondary to infective endocarditis although animal studies suggest that such therapy may reduce vegetation size and systemic embolization.

Further reading

Anguera I, Del Rio A, Moreno A, *et al.* (2006). Complications of native and prosthetic valve infective endocarditis: update in 2006. *Curr Infect Dis Rep*, 8(4), 280–8.

Habib G (2006). Management of infective endocarditis. *Heart*, 92(1), 124–30.

Hart RG, Boop BS and Anderson DC (1995). Oral anticoagulants and intracranial haemorrhage. Facts and hypotheses. *Stroke;* 26:1471–1477.

Hart RG, Foster JW, Lutherx MF and Kanter MC (1990). Stroke in infective endocarditis. *Stroke;* 21:695–700.

Kanter MC and Hart RG (1991). Neurologic complications of infective endocarditis. *Neurology;* 41:1015–1020.

Mylonakis E, Calderwood SB (2001). Infective endocarditis in adults. *NEJM;* 345:1318–1330.

Solenski NJ, Haley EC Jr (1997): Neurological complications of infective endocarditis. p 331. In Roos KL (ed): *Central Nervous System Infectious Diseases and Therapy;* Marcel Dekker, New York.

Case 26

A 45-year-old academic became anxious following a minor computational error at work. Despite reassurance, the anxiety continued for the next 9 days and was accompanied by difficulty sleeping. On the tenth day, he had difficulty accessing the computer and started to behave oddly, being unusually friendly to colleagues. Later the same day, he became sweaty and agitated and was admitted to hospital. There was no past medical history and no family history. He was on no medication, did not smoke, and took minimal alcohol.

On examination, there was no abnormality other than agitation. White cell count was 18×10^9/L with a neutrophil leucocytosis but other investigations including metabolic screen, MRI brain scan, LP, and CSF examination were normal. Over the next 3 days he exhibited episodes of odd behaviour in which he would take up specific postures and exhibit repetitive stereotyped movements, such as assuming a boxing position and executing repeated jabbing movements with his arms. In between such episodes, he displayed continuous purposeless movement and seemed excited. This was followed over the next 2 days by a gradual decrease in level of consciousness and spontaneous movements and then by the onset of rigidity. He became stuporose with a pyrexia of 38.5°C, respiratory rate of 25 breaths/min, pulse 120 beats/min, and BP 170/100 mmHg. His eyes were open but there was no blinking. There was no focal neurological abnormality but there was increased tone in the limbs with brisk reflexes. Repeat MRI brain imaging, LP and CSF examination and EEG were all normal.

Questions

26a) What is the diagnosis?

26b) How would you confirm the diagnosis?

27c) What is the prognosis?

28d) What underlying disorders are associated with this diagnosis?

29e) What is the proposed mechanism of this disorder?

30f) What is the treatment?

Answers

26a) The diagnosis is **malignant catatonia.**

The prodromal history of altered behaviour followed by pyrexia, confusion and depressed conscious level could indicate a **CNS infection (encephalitis)** or an encephalopathy. However, the brain imaging, CSF findings, blood screen and EEG were normal, making these diagnoses unlikely. **Neuroleptic malignant syndrome** and **serotonin syndrome** may produce a similar clinical picture but there was no history of any medication being taken. **Non-convulsive status** (see page 186) may produce odd behaviour and a stuporose state sometimes resembling catatonia but the EEG was normal. **Migraine coma** may present with confusion, depressed conscious level and pyrexia (see page 203) with normal investigations, but there was no history of migraine or family history in this patient, and one would not expect rigidity or the other neuropsychiatric features. **Wilson's disease** (see page 215) should be considered in anyone under the age of 55 years with a movement disorder but the presentation here is very acute. **Huntington's chorea** may cause a Parkinsonian movement disorder but again one would not expect such an acute onset. Encephalitis lethargica shares similar features to those described in this case in that sufferers become sleepy and unresponsive with an associated increase in muscle tone. Encephalitis lethargica occurred as an epidemic at the beginning of the twentieth century but this disease is now rarely, if ever, seen.

The syndrome of **catatonia** was first described by Kahlbaum in 1874 in association with either stupor or excitement and was thought to be a manifestation solely of primary psychiatric illness, particularly schizophrenia. More recently, it has become clear that it is associated most commonly with mood disorder, particularly mania, but may also occur as a result of general medical and neurological diseases. Catatonia is defined by the presence of specific motor abnormalities together with changes in thought, mood, and vigilance (see the next page for DSM criteria of which two must be present). Kahlbaum described 17 signs, but at least 40 phenomena have since been described, of which mutism, posturing, negativism, staring, rigidity, and echophenomena are the most common.

Diagnostic criteria for schizophrenia, catatonic type (DSM IV)

A type of schizophrenia* in which the clinical picture is dominated by at least two of the following:

1) Motoric immobility as evidenced by catalepsy (including waxy flexibility) or stupor.

2) Excessive motor activity (that is apparently purposeless and not motivated by external stimuli).

3) Extreme negativism (an apparently motiveless resistance to all instructions or maintenance of a rigid posture against attempts to be moved) or mutism.

4) Peculiarities of voluntary movement as evidenced by posturing (voluntary assumption of inappropriate or bizarre postures), stereotyped movements, prominent mannerisms, or prominent grimacing.

5) Echolalia or echopraxia.

   After recovery from an episode of catatonia, patients often describe a feeling of intense anxiety and fear before the attack.

   In malignant catatonia there is acute onset excitement, delirium, fever, autonomic instability, and catalepsy. The features described in this case are typical, with anxiety preceeding the onset of purposeless stereotyped movements followed by descent into stupor with increased tone, fever, tachycardia and hypertension. Malignant catatonia may be indistinguishable from neuroleptic malignant syndrome and the serotonin syndrome except for the gastrointestinal features of the latter. These drug-induced syndromes are hypothesized by some authors to represent severe forms of catatonia and the treatment is the same. Malignant hyperthermia, an autosomal dominant transmitted muscle sensitivity to inhalation anaesthetics, also shares many clinical features with malignant catatonia and has been associated with neuroleptic malignant syndrome.

26b) The diagnosis of catatonia is made on the basis of the characteristic clinical features and the exclusion of alternative diagnoses. EEG is not encephalopathic showing a responsive wakeful pattern and caloric stimulation provokes nystagmus.

26c) Malignant catatonia has a 50–70% mortality from cardiorespiratory arrest if untreated. The prognosis in milder forms of catatonia depend on the underlying diagnosis.

---

*DSM IV also recognizes that catatonia may occur with affective disorders and organic disease.

26d) Conditions associated with malignant catatonia include:

- Mood disorder, primarily mania, but also bipolar disorder and depression
- Schizophrenia
- Systemic illness e.g. autoimmune disease, metabolic disturbances, endocrinopathies, viral infections (including HIV), typhoid fever, heat stroke
- Neurological disorders e.g. Parkinsonism, multiple sclerosis, postencephalitic states, bilateral globus pallidus disease, thalamic/parietal lesions, extrapontine myelinolysis
- Drugs e.g. neuroleptics (see above), benzodiazepine withdrawal, opiate intoxication, dopaminergic drugs, recreational drugs.

26e) The mechanism of catatonia is uncertain but probably involves modulation of frontal/basal ganglia neural loops.

Parallels have been noted between the motor abnormalities of catatonia (akinesia, rigidity, posturing, waxy flexibility) and those of Parkinson's disease (bradykinesia, initiation difficulties). It has been proposed that modulation of corticosubcortical neural loops is important in both conditions. In catatonia, there is evidence for deficits in orbitofrontal (GABA-ergic) function and it has been proposed that there is subsequent 'top down' modulation of orbitofrontal/basal ganglia motor loops involved in movement control. Modulation of horizontal cortical loops specifically between orbitofrontal and right posterior inferior parietal cortex have been proposed as mediating the deficits in awareness of one's own body in space (lack of awareness of posturing and inability to terminate movement). In Parkinson's disease there is 'bottom up' modulation of subcortical/cortical motor loops resulting from a primary subcortical (substantia nigra) deficit. Recently, a genetic locus for hereditary episodic catatonia has been found on chromosome 15.

26f) Treatment is with benzodiazepines.

Initial treatment is with benzodiazepines to which approximately 70% of patients with malignant catatonia will respond. If this is ineffective, ECT may be used to good effect. Antipsychotics may worsen catatonia and precipitate the malignant form. The patient described in this case made a dramatic response to benzodiazepines, 'waking up' almost immediately but went on to develop bipolar disorder.

Further reading

Carroll BT, Anfinson TJ, Kennedy JC, Yendrek R, Boutros M, Bilon A (1994). Catatonic disorder due to general medical conditions. *J Neuropsychiatry Clin Neurosci;* 6(2):122–133.

Clark T, Richards H (1999). Catatonia. 1: History and clinical features. *Hosp Med;* 60(10):740–742. Review.

Clark T, Richards H (1999). Catatonia. 2: Diagnosis, management and prognosis. *Hosp Med;* 60(11):812–814. Review.

Fink M (2001). Catatonia: syndrome or schizophrenia subtype? Recognition and treatment. *J Neural Transm;* 108(6):637–644. Review.

Kipps CM, Fung VS, Grattar-Smith P, *et al.* (2005). Movement disorder emergencies. *Mov. Disord;* 20:322–334.

Northoff G (2002). What catatonia can tell us about 'top down modulation': a neuropsychiatric hypothesis. *Behav Brain Sci;* 25(5):555–577.

Case 27

A 85-year-old man was admitted having had a fall preceded by a sudden onset of dizziness and loss of balance. After the fall, he had been unable to get up as he felt as though the room was spinning and had recurrent vomiting. On arrival in the emergency department, he felt a little better although he was still unsteady and was drowsy. There was a past medical history of atrial fibrillation and hypertension. He was taking sotalol, warfarin, bendrofluazide and isosorbide mononitrate. He was living with his wife, was usually independent, was an ex-smoker and took little alcohol.

On examination, he was drowsy (GCS 14/15) but rousable with normal speech and swallow. Pupils were equal and reactive. There was rotatory nystagmus on upgaze and horizontal diplopia on left lateral gaze but the rest of the cranial nerve examination was normal. In the limbs, there was past pointing in the left arm. Power, tone and reflexes were normal and the plantar reflexes were downgoing. He was unable to walk because of unsteadiness. Pulse was 80/min irregularly irregular, BP 170/110mmHg, and oxygen saturation was 99% on air.

Investigations showed:

- Hb 14.5g/dL, WCC 7.7×10^9/L, plt 192×10^9/L.
- Na 139mmol/L, K 3.1mmol/L, urea 6.9mmol/L, Cr 82μmol/L.
- INR 2.6.
- CT brain is shown in Fig. 27.1.

Questions

27a) What does the CT scan (Fig. 27.1) show?

27b) What is the most common cause, seen as a contributing cause in this patient? Give 3 other causes.

27c) Of which complication is this patient at high risk? How does this affect the prognosis?

27d) How would you manage this patient?

27e) How does the management of supratentorial manifestations of this condition differ from your answer in 27d)?

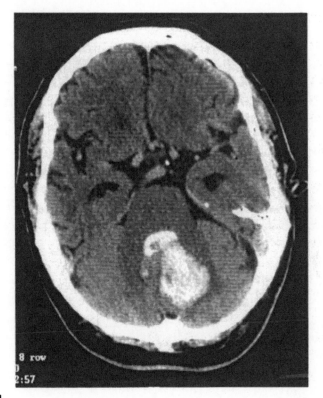

Fig. 27.1

Answers

27a) The CT scan shows **left cerebellar haemorrhage.**

There is an extensive haematoma of the cerebellum (left hemisphere and vermis), probably originating in the left sided nuclei. There is extension of blood into the IV ventricle. The basal brain arteries, especially the basilar, were considerably dilated (image not shown) in keeping with a history of hypertension.

The most frequent symptoms in cerebellar haemorrhage are headache and unsteadiness of gait, although limb ataxia, vertigo, vomiting, visual disturbance and dysarthria are also common. On examination, disturbance of level of consciousness, nystagmus, eye movement abnormalities and limb and gait ataxia are seen. For brain haemorrhage in general, mortality is greatly increased when there is intraventricular extension of blood. In cerebellar haemorrhage, mortality is around 75% versus 17% for patients with and without coma respectively.

27b) The most common cause of cerebellar haemorrhage is hypertension.

Spontaneous brain haemorrhages caused by hypertension occur most commonly in the basal ganglia, pons and cerebellum. Other causes of cerebellar haemorrhage include anticoagulants and coagulopathies, arteriovenous malformation, metastatic tumour, cavernoma and trauma.

27c) This patient is at high risk of hydrocephalus.

Patients with large cerebellar haemorrhages (>3cm) are at high risk of developing hydrocephalus and brainstem compression. This leads to rapid deterioration in conscious level and a fatality rate of 75–100%.

27d) Management of this patient includes:

- Correction of INR
- Urgent neurosurgical referral.

It is vital to instigate the correct management of patients with cerebellar haemorrhage as soon as possible, owing to the high risk of hydrocephalus and brainstem compression. It should be noted that patients may present with relatively minor symptoms and that distinguishing haemorrhage from infarction is unreliable clinically. Thus, urgent CT scanning is indicated in all patients presenting with symptoms and signs of cerebellar stroke even in those whose symptoms appear mild.

In this patient, the effects of prior warfarinization should be corrected using intravenous vitamin K. Surgical intervention is indicated for cerebellar haemorrhages greater than 3 cm diameter with neurological deterioration, brainstem compression or hydrocephalus. Surgical options comprise haematoma evacuation or insertion of a ventricular drain following which management on a neurosurgical intensive care unit is often required.

The management of blood pressure in the immediate post-stroke period is controversial since there are few randomized trials. However, aggressive blood pressure lowering should be avoided as it may cause extension of brain damage through a reduction in cerebral perfusion.

Other medical treatments that have been proposed for treatment of primary intracerbral haemorrhage include agents promoting haemostasis in view of the fact that enlargement of haematomas in the few hours after onset is common. One such agent is factor VIIa that plays a role in haemostasis after vascular injury. There is evidence that recombinant activated factor VIIa, if given within 3 hours of stroke onset, reduces haematoma growth and improves patient outcome.

27e) Surgery for supratentorial haemorrhage is controversial.

There have been a number of randomized trials and meta-analyses that have shown conflicting results. Patients in the relatively large STICH trial with haematomas of greater than 2 centimetres in diameter and GCS of 5 or greater were randomized to early surgery or conservative treatment with later surgery allowed if it was felt to be indicated by the clinical team. There was no significant benefit for early surgery although there was a trend towards benefit in those with superficial as opposed to deep haematomas, possibly related to the fact that evacuating such haematomas was likely to produce less trauma. Patients with GCS of 8 or less did uniformly badly and there was a suggestion that surgery increased the likelihood of poor outcome in this group.

Further reading

Mayer SA, Brun NC, Begtrup K *et al* (2005). Recombinant activated factor VIIa for acute intracerebral haemorrhage. *N Engl J Med*; 352:777–785.

Mendelow AD, Gregson BA, Fernandes HM *et al* (2005). Early surgery versus initial conservative treatment in patients with spontaneous supratentorial intracerebral haematomas in the International Surgical Trial in Intracerebral Haemorrhage (STICH): a randomised trial. *Lancet*; 365(9457):387–397.

Case 28

An 84-year-old woman was admitted as an emergency to the physicians via her GP. Three weeks earlier she had had a fall following which she experienced lower lumbar back pain but had been able to walk normally. Two days later she developed difficulty getting up from a sitting position and the lower back pain continued. She had long-standing urinary incontinence and constipation, which remained unchanged. There were no sensory symptoms and her symptoms were not felt to be progressing. There was a history of hypertension and hypothyroidism and she was taking aspirin, amlodipine and thyroxine. She was a non-smoker but drank upwards of 60 units of alcohol per week. She lived with her husband.

On examination, she looked well, temperature was 35.5°C, pulse 84/min regular, and blood pressure 160/80 mmHg and general systems were unremarkable. Cranial nerves were normal. Upper limb examination revealed absent biceps jerks, supinator jerk inversion and brisk triceps jerks but normal tone, power and sensation. The legs were mildly wasted proximally and there were a few calf fasciculations. There was a slight reduction in proximal leg power (hip flexion and knee extension bilaterally) but distal power was full. Knee and ankle jerks were absent. Plantar responses were flexor. Vibration sense was reduced to the knees, other sensory modalities were intact. Anal tone and sensation were normal. Her gait was unsteady and she had difficulty swinging her legs up onto the bed. She was unable to get up off the floor after falling.

Her symptoms improved over the next 2 weeks although she continued to experience lumbar back pain and her inflammatory markers remained moderately elevated. Then her mobility deteriorated suddenly with a reduction in hip flexion bilaterally to 2/5 and she developed olecranon bursitis. She became confused, although remaining apyrexial and her inflammatory markers rose to CRP>285mg/L, ESR 125mm/h and WCC 17.3×10^9/L.

Questions

28a) What is the cause of her sudden deterioration?

28b) Her symptoms and signs cannot be explained by one lesion. What is the most likely combination of processes in this patient?

28c) What investigation would you perform to confirm the cause of her sudden deterioration?

28d) How would you treat this patient?

Answers

28a) The cause of her deterioration is an **epidural abscess and discitis at L2–4.**

Fever and spinal pain followed by leg weakness are cardinal signs of an epidural abscess. Fever and pain may precede neurological symptoms by many days and, in chronic cases, weight loss and systemic upset may dominate the clinical picture. The infective source is usually cutaneous or mucosal with a posteriorly-located epidural abscess arising secondary to haematogenous spread of infection. Anteriorly located abscesses are more common as a result of direct spread of infection from the vertebral body or disc. The space around the spinal cord is small, so even very small volumes of pus may cause compressive symptoms and progression may be rapid. The most common causative organism is *Staphyloccus aureus* but *Mycobacterium tuberculosis*, *Streptococcus milleri* and Gram negative organisms are also seen and fungal infection may occur in the immunocompromised patient.

In this patient, the back pain, leg weakness and elevated inflammatory markers make an epidural abscess/discitis very likely, and the presence of an olecranon bursitis suggests septicaemia with seeding to secondary sites (see page 240). The weak hip flexion implies an L2 lesion and the absent lower limb reflexes could be secondary to a lateral cauda equina lesion affecting L2–S1 nerve roots. The lack of bladder and bowel involvement suggests sparing of the sacral roots which are affected early in a central cauda equina lesion.

28b) The clinical findings suggest multifocal pathology of the nervous system.

The absent biceps jerks with brisk triceps jerks suggest a lesion at the level of C5,6 causing a lower motor neuron abnormality with upper motor neuron signs below at the C7 level. Such lesions may cause radicular pain at the level of the lesion or a sensory level. If this were the only lesion, one would expect brisk lower limb reflexes, upgoing plantars and possibly sensory changes in the legs. There may or may not be bladder or bowel involvement. The commonest cause of such a lesion in an elderly woman would be cervical myelopathy secondary to spondylosis/canal stenosis which typically causes purely motor symptoms without bladder or bowel involvement. Absent vibration sense may be a feature.

As discussed earlier, this patient suffered an epidural abscess causing back pain and weakness of hip flexion and knee extension together with absent knee reflexes. The history of high alcohol intake may have contributed to the proximal weakness, loss of ankle jerks, and absent

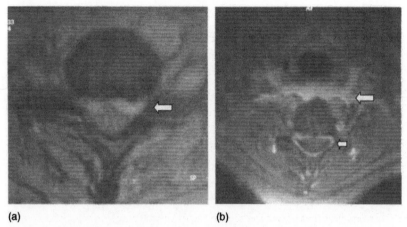

(a)   (b)

Fig. 28.1 MRI cervical spine from another patient: fat suppressed T1-weighted axial slice (left) showing bright signal between the cord and the vertebral body (epidural abscess) and fat suppressed T1-weighted gadolinium enhanced scan (right) showing high signal extra-spinally (large arrow) and around the cord (small arrow).

vibration sense seen in the legs. Calf fasciculations may occur in normal people, especially in older patients.

28c) Urgent MR (with gadolinium) imaging of the spine is required (see Fig. 28.1).

The prognosis of epidural abscess depends on the clinical condition of the patient and the time to treatment and therefore rapid imaging is mandatory once the diagnosis is suspected. Contrast MRI should be performed as this has greater sensitivity compared to plain MRI for epidural abscess. Mortality from epidural abscess is around 14% overall and is increased with diagnostic delay. In this patient, MRI spine showed an epidural abscess with L2–L4 discitis and bilateral psoas abscesses. Additional investigations included aspiration of the olecranon bursa, blood and urine cultures, and transoesophageal echocardiography to look for evidence of endocarditis. Blood and urine cultures grew methicillin resistant *Staphylococcus aureus* (MRSA) and the echocardiogram showed vegetations on the mitral valve. It was felt that the discitis/epidural abscess had been the cause of her symptoms from the outset and that this had spread to involve the heart and the bursa.

28d) Treatment of epidural abscess is with parenteral antibiotics (in this case vancomycin and gentamicin) and surgical decompression with spinal stabilization.

Further reading

Berger JR, Sabet A (2002). Infectious myelopathies. *Semin Neurol.* **22**(2):133–142. Review.

Bluman EM, Palumbo MA, Lucas PR (2004). Spinal epidural abscess in adults. *J Am Acad Orthop Surg;* **12**(3):155–163. Review.

McKenzie AR, Laing RB, Smith CC *et al* (1998). Spinal epidural abscess: the importance of early diagnosis and treatment. *J Neurol Neurosurg Psychiatry;* **65**(2):209–212. Review.

Pilkington SA, Jackson SA, Gillett GR (2003). Spinal epidural empyema. *Br J Neurosurg;* **17**(2):196–200. Review.

Case 29

A 34-year-old bricklayer was admitted with sudden-onset right-sided weakness. He had had memory problems and confusion for the preceding 3 months and had twice been found wandering disorientated in the street by neighbours. There was a past medical history of 2 strokes, 5 and 7 months earlier, the first causing right facial weakness and expressive dysphasia and the second causing expressive dysphasia, acalculia, right/left confusion and right upper limb weakness, and apraxia. CT brain after the first stroke had shown 2 small lacunar strokes in the left hemisphere in the internal capsule and anterior to the trigone.

He lived with his wife and was a smoker of 20 cigarettes a day. He drank around 20 units of alcohol per week. Medication since the first stroke was aspirin, dipyridamole, and simvastatin. There was no family history of stroke or other neurological disorder.

On examination, he appeared apathetic and withdrawn. His MMSE was 22/30, with difficulties with recall, concentration and calculation. Temperature was 36.4°C, pulse was 80/min regular and BP 100/75 mmHg. Cardiovascular examination, including for carotid bruits, was unremarkable, as was the rest of the general examination, including the skin and the eyes. There was mild upper motor neuron right facial weakness and right upper and lower limb weakness. Tendon reflexes were brisker on the right and the right plantar reflex was extensor.

Investigations showed:

- Hb 14.2 g/dL, WCC 16.3 × 10^9/L (81% neutrophils), plt 253 × 10^9/L
- CRP 9mg/L, ESR 17mm/h
- U&E, LFT, Ca, and PO$_4$ were normal
- ANA, ANCA, immunoglobulins, serum electrophoresis, hep B and C serology, complement, rheumatoid factor, ANA, ENA, lupus anticoagulant, antiphospholipid antibody, homocysteine, and cryoglobulins were all negative
- Urine dipstick and microscopy: no protein or blood, no casts seen, 24-hour collection unremarkable
- CXR and ECG: normal
- Transoesophageal echo: normal
- CSF: opening pressure 16 cm H$_2$O, glucose 3.4mmol/L (4.5mmol/L blood), protein 0.53g/L, red cells 116/mm^3, white cells 4 lymphocytes/mm^3, Gram stain negative, oligoclonal bands negative. There was no growth and no malignant cells seen.

MRI brain and cerebral angiogram from the current admission are shown in Figs. 29.1 and 29.2 respectively.

Questions

29a) What does the MRI show? What do the arrows indicate on the angiogram?

29b) What is the most likely diagnosis given the investigation results and why?

29b) How else may this condition present?

29c) What other diagnoses would you have considered?

29d) What further investigation would you request? Is this a diagnostic test?

29e) What treatment would you give?

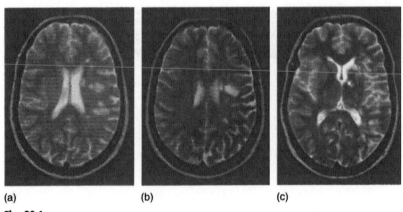

(a)   (b)   (c)

Fig. 29.1

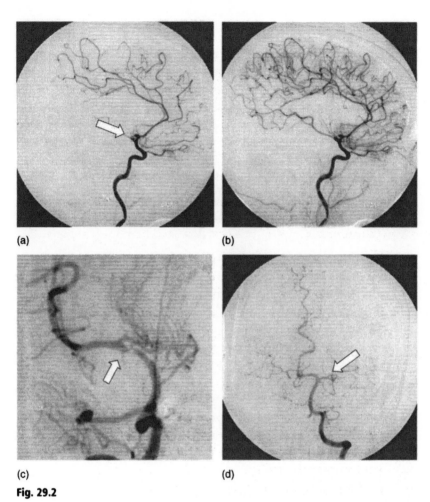

(a)

(b)

(c)

(d)

Fig. 29.2

Answers

29a) The MRI (T2-weighted) (Fig. 29.1) shows hyperintense areas in the left hemisphere in the territory supplied by the carotid artery consistent with multiple infarcts. The cerebral angiogram (Fig. 29.2) of the left internal carotid (a) shows failure of filling initially of the left MCA with subsequent perfusion via collaterals from the anterior cerebral artery (b). The angiogram of the right internal carotid artery shows distal right carotid stenosis (c). The left vertebral angiogram (d) shows failure of filling of the left posterior cerebral artery.

29b) The most likely diagnosis is **isolated CNS vasculitis** (isolated angiitis, giant cell granulomatous angiitis, cerebral granulomatous angiitis of the CNS).

This young man suffered 3 stroke-like episodes over a period of less than a year, accompanied by the onset of cognitive impairment affecting several functional domains. The clinical examination and investigations showed no evidence of a systemic vasculitis but the neuroimaging suggested multiple abnormalities of the medium sized cerebral vessels together with evidence of infarction affecting both hemispheres. This is consistent with cerebral vasculitis confined to the intracerebral vessels.

The diagnosis of isolated CNS vasculitis is difficult owing to its rarity, variety of clinical presentations, and non-specific investigation results. The following criteria have been proposed:

• Association of headaches and multiple neurological deficits persisting for at least 6 months

• Segmental arterial stenoses on cerebral angiography

• Exclusion of infectious/inflammatory causes

• Positive biopsy or exclusion of all other causes of cerebral vasculitis.

The aetiology and pathogenesis of isolated CNS vasculitis is not understood. The vascular inflammation is chronic and granulomatous affecting small and medium sized arteries and veins, particularly the leptomeningeal vessels. There is no predilection for bifurcations as in **polyarteritis nodosa** (see page 289) and eosinophils are not present in large numbers as in **Churg–Strauss** (see page 288).

Laboratory investigations are generally unremarkable in isolated CNS vasculitis and the aim is to exclude alternative diagnoses (see below for the causes of CNS vasculitis). The ESR may be raised (in about 30% of autopsy confirmed cases) but not to the extent seen in temporal arteritis. Specific CNS investigations are usually non-specific. The CSF may show a pleocytosis, elevated protein and occasionally a low glucose but may be normal. Oligoclonal bands are rare.

CT has poor sensitivity (around 30%) but may show multiple focal areas of low intensity and sometimes haemorrhage together with focal cerebral atrophy and multiple areas of parenchymal enhancement. MRI has greater sensitivity (around 80%) particularly for small lesions, and there may be widespread T2-weighted hyperintensity indicating leukoencephalopathy (see page 84). Linear and punctate patterns of leptomeningeal enhancement associated with both hemispheric and penetrating vessels may occur even in the absence of significant parenchymal abnormality. Unusual appearances have been reported including appearances suggestive of tumour or demyelination. MRA is being used increasingly as the first line investigation of the intracerebral vessels but it has low sensitivity for abnormalities of the smaller cerebral vessels.

29c) Isolated CNS vasculitis may present with:

- Headache
- Encephalopathy
- Focal neurological deficit
- Seizures.

The mode of onset in isolated CNS vasculitis is acute or subacute and the most common presentation is with headache and confusion with or without focal neurological deficit, most commonly hemiparesis. Ataxia, aphasia and seizures are also frequent, and almost every neurological symptom and sign has been reported. Classically there is progressive multifocal and cumulative neurological dysfunction. However, the presentation can mimic dementia, demyelinating disease, tumour, encephalitis and chronic meningitis. All types of stroke including SAH have been reported and although stroke may be the presenting feature, it occurs typically on a background of diffuse cerebral symptoms. Systemic symptoms are generally absent although fever occurs in around 15%.

29d) The differential diagnosis includes:

- Large/small vessel atherosclerosis
- Systemic vasculitis
- CADASIL
- MELAS.

The differential diagnosis for isolated CNS vasculitis is often very broad as the symptoms and signs are non-specific. However, the syndrome described in this case is highly suggestive comprising recurrent stroke with cognitive impairment and a vasculitic appearance on angiography. Strokes and encephalopathy may occur in systemic vasculitides (see table below for list of causes) particularly **polyarteritis nodosa** and **Churg–Strauss** and may rarely be the presenting feature. However, the lack of supporting evidence makes a systemic vasculitis unlikely.

Although he was a smoker, recurrent stroke caused by **large vessel atherosclerosis** or **small vessel disease** would be unusual in a man of this age and one would not expect cognitive impairment or the angiographic findings. The syndrome of **CADASIL** (see page 71) causes recurrent stroke at a young age and dementia with frontal features of apathy and loss of executive function. However, there was no family history of young stroke or dementia and the imaging findings were not typical of CADASIL in which multiple subcortical and periventricular abnormalities are seen. **MELAS** (see page 103) is another inherited disorder in which there are recurrent stroke-like episodes and encephalopathy but again there was little clinically to suggest this diagnosis, and the imaging abnormalities in MELAS are typically cortical, not within defined vascular territories and often occipital. **Infective endocarditis** is an important cause of stroke (see page 150), particularly in the young, and may be associated with encephalopathy, but there was no evidence to support this; the history was rather long and cognitive impairment would be unusual. **Hashimoto's encephalitis** (see page 98) causes stroke-like episodes and encephalopathy but one would not expect the imaging changes seen in this case.

Causes of cerebral vasculitis

- *Infectious*:
  - Viral e.g. varicella/herpes zoster, CMV, HIV
  - Fungal e.g. aspergillosis
  - Bacterial e.g. syphilis, *Borrelia burgdorferi*, TB, bacterial meningitis.
- *Primary systemic vasculitis*:
  - Necrotizing e.g. PAN, Churg–Strauss, microscopic polyangiitis
  - Giant cell e.g. temporal arteritis, Takayasu's arteritis

- Granulomatous e.g. Wegener's, lymphomatoid
- Other e.g. Buerger's, Kawasaki's arteritis.

- *Vasculitis secondary to systemic disease*:
  - SLE, rheumatoid arthritis, Sjogren's, scleroderma
  - Behçet's
  - Sarcoid
  - Dermatomyositis
  - Ulcerative colitis
  - Coeliac disease.

- *Associated with neoplasia*:
  - Hodgkin's/non-Hodgkin's lymphoma
  - Hairy cell leukaemia
  - Malignant histiocytosis.

- *Associated with drugs*:
  - Cocaine, amphetamines
  - Sympathomimetic agents.

- *Isolated CNS vasculitis.*

29e) Cerebral angiography should be performed but is not diagnostic.

Angiography may be normal (up to 50%) even in pathologically documented cases particularly when small vessels (<500μm in diameter) only are involved. Alternatively, widespread segmental changes in the contour and calibre of the vessels and small aneurysms may be seen. However, even the angiographic abnormalities are non specific: similar changes may be seen in MELAS, reversible cerebral vasoconstriction, infective endocarditis and atrial myxoma (the latter two conditions being associated with small aneurysms). Definitive diagnosis is achieved with brain-leptomeningeal biopsy although false negatives may occur.

29f) Immunosuppressive treatment should be considered.

There are no randomized controlled trials of therapy in isolated CNS vasculitis. There are data from non-randomized comparisons suggesting that treatment with steroids or steroids and cyclophosphamide leads to a favourable outcome, whereas lack of treatment is associated with rapid progression to death or to severe deficits. However, earlier case series may have been biased towards more severely affected patients and there is some evidence that the prognosis in isolated CNS vasculitis is not uniformly poor. Aggressive immunosuppressive treatment should probably be reserved for those patients who show continuing deterioration or severe complications such as stroke.

Further reading

Calabrese LH, Duna GF and Lie JT (1997). Vasculitis in the central nervous system. *Arth Rheum;* **40**:1189–1201.

Moore PM (1998). Central nervous system vasculitis. *Curr Opin Neurol;* **11**:241-246.

Vollmer TL, Guarnaccia J, Harrington W *et al* (1993). Idiopathic granulomatous angiitis of the central nervous system:diagnostic challenges. *Arch Neurol;* **50**:925–930.

Case 30

Case A A 50-year-old schizophrenic woman was admitted from a local psychiatric hospital following several generalized tonic clonic seizures. There was no past history of epilepsy and she had been well prior to the seizures. She was taking chlorpromazine. On admission she was unresponsive with a Glasgow Coma Scale (GCS) score of 6. Her eyes were deviated to the left and there was an apparent right facial weakness. Tone was increased, there was flexion to pain in all 4 limbs and the plantar responses were extensor. Temperature, pulse, and blood pressure were normal.

Investigations revealed Na 110mmol/L, K 2.9mmol/L, chloride 72mmol/L, urea 2.9mmol/L and glucose 12.1mmol/L. Serum osmolality was 233mosm/kg (278–305mosm/kg) and urine osmolality was 87mosm/kg (350–1000mosmol/kg).

Case B A 44-year-old chronic schizophrenic man was admitted from a local psychiatric hospital after 3 generalized tonic-clonic seizures. There was no past history of epilepsy. Medications comprised thioridazine and haloperidol. On admission, he was unresponsive with a GCS score of 5, marked neck stiffness, dysconjugate eye movements and bilateral papilloedema. There was no motor response in the right arm or leg, but extension to pain on the left side. Tone was increased in all limbs and both plantar responses were extensor. He was afebrile with normal pulse and blood pressure.

Investigations revealed Na 107mmol/L, chloride 68mmol/L, potassium 3.3mmol/L, urea 1.3mmol/L and glucose 6.7mmol/L. Serum osmolality was 226mosm/kg and urine osmolality was 189mosm/kg. CT brain and CSF were normal.

Case C A 28-year-old woman was admitted following a collapse. One week previously she had had a skin biopsy, since which time she had been very anxious. On admission she was unrousable with a GCS score of 7, but was moving all limbs and had no localizing signs or papilloedema. She was afebrile and pulse and blood pressure were normal.

Investigations revealed Na 119mmol/L, K 3.6mmol/L, urea 1.8mmol/L and glucose 6.8mmol/L. A CT brain scan and CSF were normal.

Questions

30a) What is the diagnosis applicable to all the cases?

30b) Which patient characteristics are associated with this diagnosis?

30c) What neurological abnormalities may be associated with a low serum sodium and what is the significance of seizures?

30d) How would you treat these patients?

30e) What complication of treatment is shown on the MRI in Fig. 30.1?

30f) What are the clinical features of the diagnosis in 30e) and with which 2 conditions is it particularly associated?

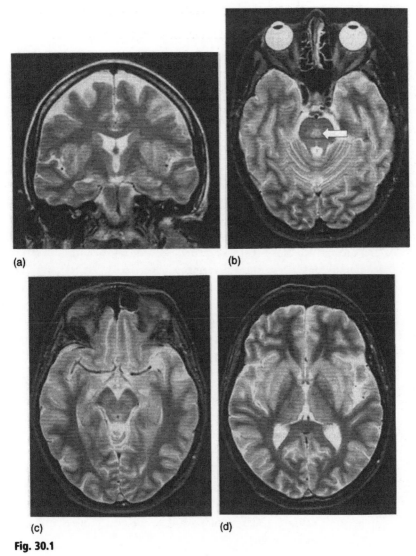

(a)

(b)

(c)

(d)

Fig. 30.1

Answers

30a) The diagnosis is **psychogenic polydipsia** (primary or hysterical polydipsia) with consequent hyponatraemia.

30b) Psychogenic polysipsia occurs in psychiatric patients, particularly those with psychosis or mania. Occasionally it is thought to be a manifestation of hypothalamic damage e.g. in neurosarcoid (see page 273).

30c) Hyponatraemia is the most common electrolyte abnormality seen in hospitalized patients.

Children and women of reproductive age are most at risk from brain damage from low serum sodium. Certain underlying causes including polydipsia, postoperative state, pharmacological agents and heart failure are also more likely to be associated with brain damage. Hyponatraemia is more likely to cause neurological deficits if the rate of change of serum sodium is rapid. In such cases, even small decreases in Na concentration e.g. to 130mmol/L may be enough to cause symptoms. In contrast, much lower levels of Na concentration may be tolerated if they have occurred gradually. Hyponatraemia, where symptomatic, most commonly causes confusion which ranges from mild to coma. EEG shows non-specific slow wave abnormalities. Focal neurological deficits (see page 136) may occur including hemiparesis, ataxia, nystagmus, tremor, and aphasia. Seizures are associated with a grave prognosis (mortality of around 50%).

30d) The management of hyponatraemia depends on the patient's fluid volume status (see page 137).

Patients with primary polydipsia are hypervolaemic and where hyponatraemia and associated symptoms are mild or absent, fluid restriction should be instituted. Active correction of hyponatraemia with hypertonic saline is controversial owing to the possibility of inducing complications (see below).

Once the patient with hyponatraemia secondary to polydipsia has been stabilized, close monitoring including daily weights and regular serum sodium is required since many patients will continue to try and drink excessively even to the extent of taking water from plant pots and toilets. Underlying psychiatric disease should be considered in those without a prior diagnosis.

30e) The T2–weighted MRI brain Fig. 30.1 shows **central pontine (arrow) and extra-pontine (basal ganglia) myelinolysis.** The most commonly associated disorders are alcoholism and malnutrition.

In central pontine myelinolysis, there is demyelination of brainstem areas centred on the basis pontis where there is extensive mixing of grey and white matter. Clinical signs of central pontine myelinolysis include dysarthria and dysphagia and quadraparesis (initially flaccid then becoming spastic). Locked in syndrome and eye movement abnormalities may occur if damage extends to the pontine tegmentum. Extra pontine myelinolysis may occur together with central pontine myelinolysis or occasionally in isolation and causes mutism, Parkinsonism, dystonia, and catatonia (see page 160).

An association between correction of hyponatraemia and central pontine myelinolysis has been known since the 1970s. Patients often go through a biphasic clinical course presenting with encephalopathy or seizures from hyponatraemia, recovering as the sodium normalizes, only to deteriorate several days later. Certain conditions including alcoholism, malnutrition, liver transplantation, prolonged diuretic use, pituitary surgery, and burns, make patients more vulnerable to central pontine myelinolysis. Of note, central pontine myelinolysis is rare in psychogenic polydipsia where the hyponatraemia has developed rapidly. It is hypothesized that cell damage occurs secondary to osmotic stress and that such damage may be more severe in patients who are malnourished or who have other conditions resulting in reduced ability of the cells to counteract the osmotic stress through synthesis of organic osmoles.

There is little data on which to guide the rate of correction of sodium in hyponatraemic patients: some patients have developed pontine myelinolysis after very slow rates of sodium rise. In general, the more rapid the development of hyponatraemia, the safer it is to correct the sodium rapidly. However, in practice, it is often unclear whether or not the low sodium is chronic. The current consensus seems to be that correction should not exceed 8–10mmol per day (this is much lower than previous suggested correction rates). In patients with seizures or severe neurological deficits, more rapid partial correction of hyponatraemia may be justified.

Further reading

Fraser CL, Arieff AI (1997). Epidemiology, pathophysiology, and management of hyponatremic encephalopathy. *Am J Med*; **102**(1):67–77.

Martin RJ (2004). Central pontine and extrapontine myelinolysis: the osmotic demyelination syndromes. *J Neurol Neurosurg Psychiatry*; **75** Suppl 3:iii22–28.

Kubacki A (1989). Psychogenic polydipsia revisited. *Am J Psychiatry*; **146**(9):1235.

Smith DM, McKenna K, Thompson CJ (2003). Hyponatraemia. *Clin Endocrinol (Oxf)*; **59**(1):142.

Case 31

A 33-year-old female librarian was brought by her husband to the emergency department with odd behaviour. She had been well until 2 days previously but since that time had been wandering about the house in an apparently confused state, staring blankly, and not replying to her husband's questions. There was a past medical history of epilepsy beginning during eclampsia associated with her second pregnancy 6 years earlier. Her seizures were usually generalized motor seizures but sometimes she would become vague or experience déjà vu. Her epilepsy had been difficult to control initially but over the 6 months prior to the time of presentation in the emergency department, she had had about 1 seizure a month. She had developed mild memory and more general cognitive impairment since the onset of her epilepsy. Her antiepileptic medication comprised sodium valproate and lamotrigine, which had remained unchanged for over a year. Fluoxetine had recently been prescribed by her GP for depression.

On examination, she was pyrexial at 37.8°C, with a pulse of 90 regular, and blood pressure of 130/70 mmHg. General systems examination was normal and there was no neck stiffness or photophobia. She replied intermittently and occasionally appropriately to questions but appeared restless and disorientated with a blank, staring aspect. Examination of the cranial nerves and limbs was normal. Her gait was normal.

Investigations showed:

- FBC, U&E, glc, LFT, TFT all normal
- CRP 15g/L, ESR 30.

Questions

31a) What is the most likely diagnosis and why?

31b) Which other conditions may this disorder mimic?

31c) What other investigation would you request to confirm your diagnosis? Is this investigation always diagnostic?

31d) What factor might have contributed to the development of this problem in this patient?

31e) How would you treat this patient and what is the prognosis in this condition?

Answers

31a) The most likely diagnosis is **focal non convulsive status epilepticus** (NCSE) (complex partial status or temporal lobe status).

Non convulsive status epilepticus is characterized by behavioural or cognitive change from baseline for at least 30 minutes with EEG evidence of seizures. Non-convulsive status epilepticus is not uncommon, accounting for at least one quarter of all cases of status epilepticus. Seizure activity may be generalized (primary or secondary) or focal.

This patient has a history of epilepsy together with episodes of déjà vu, memory and cognitive impairment suggesting that the epileptic focus is in the temporal lobe(s). Temporal lobe seizures may cause a variety of sensory symptoms including olfactory and auditory hallucinations, emotional or psychic symptoms or autonomic symptoms. Distortions of memory include dream states, flashbacks and sensations of familiarity with unfamiliar events (déjá vu) or unfamiliarity with situations previously experienced (jamais vu). Feelings of pleasure or displeasure, fear and terror, or depression and unworthiness may occur.

Complex partial seizures in which there is clouding of cognition in the absence of generalized seizure activity may occur in temporal or frontal lobe epilepsy. Such attacks present typically with altered mental status, confusion, or symptoms suggestive of psychosis and features range from semi-responsiveness and semi-purposeful automatisms (more or less coordinated, involuntary motor activity occurring during a state of impaired consciousness e.g. drinking from a cup) to total unresponsiveness with speech arrest and stereotypical automatisms. Continuous complex partial seizures or recurrent seizures with incomplete interictal recovery lead to **focal NCSE (complex partial status)**. Patients with focal NCSE may show features similar to those seen in complex partial seizures but may still be able to communicate and obey commands albeit less fluently than normal.

Generalized NCSE may occur in patients with absence seizures (absence status) and cause stupor, clouding of consciousness and little or no motor activity. Generalized NCSE may also occur in patients without absence epilepsy and cause confusion, coma or catatonic-like state. Usually, this occurs in a patient with known generalized motor seizures and often follows a motor seizure or seizures but it may also occur de novo in middle-aged and elderly patients without a past history of epilepsy and lead to diagnostic difficulties.

A high index of suspicion is required to make the diagnosis of NCSE, particularly in those without a history of seizures, since it may mimic a number of other disorders (see below). Confirmation requires an EEG, often a test not readily available out of hours or in hospitals without neurological units.

31b) Non-convulsive status may resemble:

- CNS infection e.g. herpes simplex encephalitis (see page 4)
- Psychosis
- Catatonia (see page 158).

Non-convulsive status may mimic other conditions causing clouding of consciousness with or without behavioural changes and thus any condition causing encephalopathy. In particular, CNS infection, particularly non-pyogenic infection in which acute phase responses are less marked, psychosis and catatonia are common differential diagnoses. Occasionally, focal neurological dysfunction may occur without clouding of consciousness secondary to focal NCSE in areas other than the temporal lobe. For example, expressive aphasia may result from focal NCSE affecting the frontal cortex mimicking a stroke.

31c) EEG should be performed.

When the EEG demonstrates typical ictal patterns, the diagnosis is usually straightforward. However, in many cases of NCSE, the EEG has a more encephalopathic pattern in which case the clinical and electrographic response to treatment may prove helpful. Diagnosis is often the most difficult in those with learning difficulties in whom the clinical presentation may be subtle and the diagnosis may be missed.

31d) The prescription of fluoxetine may have precipitated increased seizure frequency.

In any patient with status epilepticus, precipitating factors should be sought including the following:
- Intercurrent illness
- Metabolic abnormality
- Recent change in antiepileptic medication
- Addition of medication known to lower seizure threshold e.g. antidepressants, ciprofloxacin, or drugs interfering with the metabolism of antiepileptic medication
- Seizure secondary to a new pathology e.g. stroke.

All antidepressants lower the seizure threshold and should be prescribed with caution in patients with epilepsy. They may also interact with antiepileptic medication e.g. fluoxetine raises the plasma levels of carbamezepine and phenytoin.

31e) The prognosis in NCSE is unclear.

The prognosis is NCSE is complicated by a number of factors including underdiagnosis, incorrect diagnosis and grouping of widely disparate populations with differing comorbidities. Overall, it is likely that the underlying aetiology is the most important prognostic factor. From the available data, it appears that generalized NCSE with typical absence epilepsy does not cause lasting morbidity but that focal NCSE has varying outcome with many patients appearing to be unharmed in the long term but with others appearing to sustain memory damage. In general, NCSE does not require treatment with the same degree of urgency as convulsive SE in which neuronal damage and metabolic and respiratory derangement occur rapidly. In general, oral benzodiazepines are appropriate treatment for absence NCSE and ambulant patients with focal NCSE although intravenous medication may be required, particularly in patients with more severe impairment of consciousness. Induction of anaesthetic coma is not recommended.

Further reading

Brenner RP (2002). Is it status? *Epilepsia;* **43** Suppl 3:103–113. Review.

Chung PW, Seo DW, Kwon JC *et al* (2002). Nonconvulsive status epilepticus presenting as a subacute progressive aphasia. *Seizure;* 11(7):449–454. Review.

Kaplan PW (2000). Prognosis in nonconvulsive status epilepticus. *Epileptic Disord;* 2(4):185–193. Review.

Lee SI (1985). Nonconvulsive status epilepticus. Ictal confusion in later life. *Arch Neurol;* 42:778–781.

Walker MC (2001). Diagnosis and treatment of nonconvulsive status epilepticus. *CNS Drugs;* 15(12):931–939. Review

Case 32

A 48-year-old female bank clerk presented to the emergency department having become acutely agitated. She had become unwell earlier that day at work and had had diarrhoea and vomiting. This was followed by severe headache and agitation. There was a history of hypothyroidism and she was taking thyroxine.

On examination, the temperature was 36.5°C and there was no rash. GCS was 14/15. General systems were unremarkable. There was neck stiffness but no rash or papilloedema, a dilated right pupil and her eyes were deviated to the left. There was increased tone in the limbs with brisk reflexes and upgoing plantars.

Investigations showed:

- Hb 12.7, WCC 15.4 (14.36 neutrophils), plt 247, CRP 183, TSH 1.8
- CT with contrast: cerebral oedema only
- LP: opening pressure 36 cm H_2O, protein 1.5g/L, glucose 1.5mmol/L (blood 6.2mmol/L), 3430 white cells/mm^3 (2250 neutrophils, 1180 lymphocytes, 1860 red cells).

Questions

32a) What is the most likely diagnosis? What are the two most likely organisms?

32b) What are the neurological complications of this condition?

32c) What treatment would you give?

Treatment was commenced and she was transferred to ITU. On weaning from the ventilator, it was noted that she was unable to move her arms or legs. On examination, the cranial nerves were normal but the limbs were flaccid with power 1/5 throughout. Reflexes were brisk and the plantar reflexes were upgoing. Abdominal reflexes were absent. Pin prick was reduced to the chest but joint position sense was preserved. Anal tone was reduced and she had no sensation of opening her bowels. A urinary catheter was in situ. An MRI scan of the spine was normal.

32d) What is the specific neurological syndrome suggested by the ITU findings? Explain the neuroanatomical substrates of this syndrome.

32e) What are the possible causes in this patient? Give 3 other causes.

32f) What are the ITU-associated causes of limb weakness?

Answers

32a) The most likely diagnosis is **bacterial meningitis**. The most likely causative organisms in a patient this age are *Neisseria meningitidis* or *Streptococcus pneumoniae*.

The history of headache and agitation, neck stiffness and focal neurological signs together with neutrophilia, high CRP, cerebral oedema, and neutrophilic CSF with high protein content strongly suggest bacterial meningitis. In this case, gram stain of the CSF showed Gram negative diplococci and *N. meningitidis* was subsequently cultured. Diarrhoea and pain in the calves are features of meningococcal infection in which progression may be so rapid that the patient becomes comatose within a few hours. The rash of meningococcal infection is petechial, often appearing first on the shins or the volar aspects of the forearms. An identical rash may occur with echovirus, leptospirosis, *Staphylococcus aureus*, *Strep. pneumoniae*, *Haemophilus influenzae*, salmonella, and infections associated with infective endocarditis. The brownish red, geometrical, vasculitic rash of fulminant meningococcaemia is unmistakeable and there is associated shock, spontaneous bleeding and gangrene of the extremities.

N. meningitidis and *Strep. pneumoniae* cause 70–80% of community acquired meningitis in adults. Most of the remaining cases are caused by *Listeria monocytogenes*, aerobic Gram negative bacilli (such as *Escherichia coli*), *H. influenzae*, and *Staph. aureus*. The incidence of pneumococcal meningitis increases in those over 70 years of age and in many cases there is an associated focus such as otitis media or sinusitis. Staphylococcal meningitis is associated with infective collections elsewhere in the body (see page 240), infective endocarditis (see page 148) and neurosurgical procedures. The risks of listeria infection are increased in those at extremes of age, pregnant women and the immunosuppressed including those with AIDS (see page 227), although the use of trimethoprim-sulfamethoxazole for *Pneumocystis carinii* prophylaxis has reduced the incidence of listeria in the latter group. *E. coli* infection is more likely in the elderly, debilitated and diabetic. The rate of *H. influenza* group B has been declining owing to the introduction of the Hib vaccine. Opportunistic infections are common in the immunocompromised patient (see page 227) and require specific culture techniques, serology, and/or PCR testing.

A raised white cell count with a neutrophil predominance is typical of bacterial meningitis, although rarely counts may be normal, for example in overwhelming pneumococcal infection, or there may be a lymphocyte predominance in early infection or in opportunistic infections such as listeria. Gram stain reveals the organism in 50–80% of cases. The latex agglutination test (LA test) for the detection of bacterial antigen may be useful particularly in patients who have already received antibiotics. The LA test has high specificity for both *S. pneumoniae* and *N. meningitidis* and also detects *H. influenzae* group b, *E. coli* and group B streptococci. Sensitivity is lower however, so a negative LA test does not exclude infection. PCR tests are becoming available but are not yet fully reliable. CSF glucose is usually low (<0.31 of serum glucose). Protein is usually elevated (>1.5g/L).

The most common differential diagnosis of bacterial meningitis is **acute viral meningitis** (see page 4). In viral meningitis, the CSF typically contains a predominance of lymphocytes, glucose is normal or mildly reduced, and protein may be elevated but typically <1 g/L. Similar CSF profile is seen in opportunistic infection. Focal infection including **brain abscess, subdural empyema** (see page 258), and **epidural abscess** (see page 168) may also cause similar symptoms to those of bacterial meningitis. The presence of such a mass lesion is suggested by focal or generalized seizure activity or focal neurological deficits and should be excluded by neuroimaging. **Tuberculous meningitis** (see page 54) may present in a fulminant fashion mimicking bacterial meningitis. **Subarachnoid haemorrhage** may need to be excluded in some patients in whom the history is unclear or in whom headache onset has been sudden.

32b) The complications of bacterial meningitis are many and are caused by the effects of the subarachnoid inflammatory exudate. They include:

- Cranial neuropathy
- Vasculitis
- Subdural empyema
- CVT
- Hyponatraemia
- Seizures
- Hydrocephalus.

Cranial neuropathy, particularly sensorineural deafness together in some cases with tinnitus and vertigo from damage to the VIII nerve (VI, III, VII, and II may also be affected), is seen usually 2–9 days after symptom onset. Vascular lesions secondary to vasculitis may produce hemiparesis or quadraparesis, speech disorders, and visual field defects. Subdural effusion or empyema (see page 258) is a common complication of *H. influenzae* meningitis in children under 2-years-old. CVT (see page 10) and hydrocephalus (communicating or obstructive) (see page 240) may occur. Hyponatraemia may develop as a consequence of the syndrome of inappropriate ADH secretion. 20–40% per cent of patients develop seizures.

32c) Treatment includes:

- Empirical broad spectrum antibiotics
- Steroids
- Supportive measures.

Empirical treatment for bacterial meningitis should be started with broad spectrum antibiotics that penetrate the CNS (e.g. ceftriaxone) according to local policy together with aciclovir until bacterial infection has been confirmed. Ampicillin should be added if there is any suspicion of listeria monocytogenes. Vancomycin should be added if *Staph. aureus* is a possibility. Treatment should not be delayed until after lumbar puncture but ideally blood cultures should be taken first. Supportive therapy includes ventilatory and circulatory support in patients with reduced conscious level and or circulatory compromise and correction of electrolyte abnormalities. Measures to reduce raised intracranial pressure, including shunting for patients with hydrocephalus, may be required.

The complications of meningitis are caused by the inflammatory reaction in the subarachnoid space induced by the infection. Consequently, brain damage progresses long after the CSF has become sterile. Lysis of bacteria with the release of bacterial cell wall components is the initial step in the induction of the inflammatory process. This stimulates production of inflammatory cytokines and consequently blood brain barrier breakdown with leakage of serum proteins and other molecules into the CSF. Dexamethasone inhibits the production of TNF if administered to macrophages and microglia before they are activated by bacterial lysis. A recent systematic review concluded that adjuvant steroid therapy was associated with a significant reduction in mortality from pneumococcal meningitis and a non significant reduction in mortality and morbidity from meningococcal meningitis and thus that adjuvant steroid therapy should be started with or before the first dose of antibiotics in most patients.

32d) The neurological syndrome suggested by the ITU findings is **anterior spinal artery syndrome.**

The clinical findings of tetraparesis with a sensory level and preservation of joint position sense suggest an anterior spinal artery syndrome. The anterior part of the spinal cord is supplied by the single anterior spinal artery which runs in the ventral sulcus of the spinal cord and arises from the vertebral arteries in the foramen magnum as two vessels that join to become a single vessel opposite the odontoid peg. Various feeder vessels anastomose with the anterior cerebral artery but there is variability between individuals. There is a fairly constant vessel entering with the C3 or C4 root and originating from the thyrocervical trunk. Further feeder vessels join at the thoracic level, the most important being the arteria magna of Adamkiewicz which arises from the left T10, T11, or T12 intercostal artery in 75% of the population. Damage to this vessel causes infarction of the cord up to T3/T4 level. The posterior segment of the cord receives blood from the paired posterior spinal arteries which form a plexus.

Occlusion of the anterior spinal artery causes acute loss of power and pain and temperature sensation below the occlusion since the anterior and lateral corticospinal tracts and the spinothalamic tracts lie in the anterior and lateral parts of the cord. Vibration and position sense are carried in the dorsal columns of the spinal cord supplied by the posterior spinal artery hence these sensory modalities are not usually compromised by anterior spinal artery occlusion. The level of the lesion depends on the level at which the vascular supply is compromised: occlusion of the arteria magna usually causes damage to T4–T6 and below resulting in a flaccid paraplegia often with accompanying severe back pain. Arteriosclerosis at the origin of the vertebral arteries may occlude the origin of the anterior spinal artery and cause medullary and cervical cord infarction with flaccid tetraparesis. Lumbar feeder vessel disease may cause intermittent claudication of the cauda equina but rarely causes infarction at this level. MRI of the spine in anterior spinal artery occlusion may be normal (cf. brain imaging after ischaemic stroke) or there may be an area of T2–weighted hyperintensity.

32e) Anterior spinal artery occlusion associated with meningitis may be caused in a number of ways:

- Vasculitis of the anterior spinal artery
- Direct occlusion following infiltration by organisms (e.g. aspergillus)
- Hypotension secondary to sepsis
- Thromboembolism associated with vasculitis in remote vessels or with direct organism invasion.

Other causes include surgical procedures such as nephrectomy, lumbar sympathectomy, splenectomy and intercostal nerve block (damaging the arteria magna) or neck procedures damaging the C3/C4 feeder vessel. Aortic surgery may also compromise supply of the anterior spinal artery. Medical causes include aortic dissection see page 118, atheroma, cardioembolism, sickle cell disease, and microvascular disease secondary to diabetes, syphilis, infective endocarditis, and vasculitis e.g. polyarteritis nodosa. Recovery after anterior spinal artery occlusion is variable but almost complete resolution may occur in some patients.

32f) Causes of limb weakness associated with ITU admission are:

- Critical illness neuropathy

- Critical illness myopathy.

Limb weakness associated with ITU admission (excluding those causes that are themselves responsible for the ITU admission such as Guillain–Barré syndrome) is caused by a critical illness neuropathy or myopathy. Critical illness polyneuropathy is relatively common problem in intensive care units affecting around one-half of patients and is a predominantly axonal motor neuropathy thought to be a complication of the systemic inflammatory response. The first sign of critical illness polyneuropathy may be when there is difficulty weaning a patient from the ventilator. Limb movements are weak or absent but head, face and jaw movements are relatively well preserved. Severity of the neuropathy correlates with the length of time spent on ITU. NCS show distal axonal neuropathy with fibrillation potentials and decreased motor unit potentials on EMG. CSF is almost always normal. Myopathy may also occur in association with critical illness (see page 107). High dose corticosteroids and neuromuscular blocking agents have been implicated in some cases.

Further reading

van de Beek D, de Gans J, McIntyre P, Prasad K (2004). Steroids in adults with acute bacterial meningitis: a systematic review. *Lancet Infect Dis;* **4**(3):139–143.

Choi C (2001). Bacterial meningitis in aging adults. *Clin Infect Dis;* **33**(8):1380–1385.

Lacomis D, Giuliani MJ, Van Cott A *et al.* (1996). Acute myopathy of intensive care: clinical, electromyographic, and pathological aspects. *Ann Neurol;* **40**:645–654.

Peterman AF, Yoss RE, Corbin KB (1958). The syndrome of occlusion of the anterior spinal artery. *Proc Mayo Clin;* **33**:31.

Roos KL (2000). Acute bacterial meningitis. *Semin Neurol;* **20**(3):293–306.

Steegman AT (1952). Syndrome of the anterior spinal artery. *Neurology;* **2**:15.

Case 33

A 40-year-old man presented with a 3-week history of gradual onset diffuse headache and nausea associated with loss of concentration and memory. The headache was exacerbated by standing or sitting up and was relieved by lying down. There was no medical history, no relevant family history and he was not taking any medication.

General systems examination was normal. He was alert and orientated in place but not in time and short-term memory was poor. His long-term memory was intact and there was no other neurological abnormality.

Investigations showed:

- CT brain: unremarkable.
- LP: CSF opening pressure 4 cm H_2O, 2 lymphocytes/mm^3, protein 0.67g/L, glucose 3.3mm/L (blood glucose 5.9mm/L), no organisms or acid fast bacilli.

Questions

33a) What is the diagnosis? Describe the clinical features that may be seen in this condition.

33b) What is the most common cause of this type of headache? Give 2 further causes.

33c) How would you confirm your diagnosis and what findings would you expect?

33d) How would you treat this patient?

Answers

33a) The diagnosis is **spontaneous intracranial hypotension.**

The postural nature of the headache in the absence of other clinical symptoms or signs except poor short term memory strongly suggests a diagnosis of spontaneous intracranial hypotension resulting in low-pressure, headache.

Typically, low pressure headache is worsened by standing or sitting and relieved by lying down. However, the postural nature of the headache may become less noticeable as the condition becomes more chronic and the headache more persistent, particularly if there is secondary subdural haematoma formation. Nausea and vomiting, low back pain, tinnitus, cranial nerve palsies and upper limb sensory abnormalities may occur. Unusual features include sphincter dysfunction, progressive cognitive decline, diencephalic compression causing progressive stupor, and severe encephalopathy with seizures. The neurological abnormalities are thought to be caused by loss of the normal cushioning effect of CSF with resulting traction on the brain and cranial nerves. Occasionally intracranial hypotension can be followed by raised intracranial pressure due to the development of subdural haematomas.

33b) Causes of low pressure headache include:

- LP
- Dural tears secondary to trauma/surgery/tumour invasion
- Trauma/surgery/tumour invasion to skull base
- Spontaneous dural leak.

LP is the commonest cause of intracranial hypotension. Symptoms usually resolve after a few hours but may persist for weeks, or even months. Dural tears, usually in the mid thoracic region, may arise through major or minor trauma e.g. crush injuries to the chest or abdomen or lifting or coughing, or as a result of overdraining CSF shunts. Occasionally, CSF may be lost through the cribriform plate, petrous bones, or through a basal skull defect as a result of trauma or tumour erosion. CSF rhinorrhea or otorrhea may not be noticed by the patient who may complain of post-traumatic or spontaneous headache. However, many cases of intracranial low pressure headache appear to arise spontaneously at the level of the thoracic spine or the cervicothoracic junction.

33c) Investigation of low pressure headache involves:

- MRI
- Myelogram
- LP.

The diagnosis is made on MRI and/or myelogram (see Fig. 33.1–3 for the findings in this patient), which sometimes show leakage of

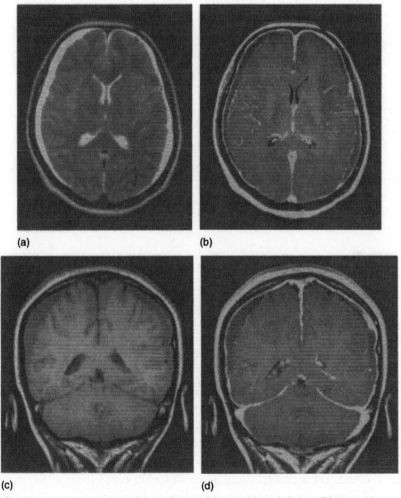

(a)

(b)

(c)

(d)

Fig. 33.1 Axial T2-weighted (a), axial T1-weighted with gadolinium (b), coronal T1-weighted (c) and coronal T1-weighted with gadolinium (d) MRI showing subdural effusions and meningeal thickening and enhancement.

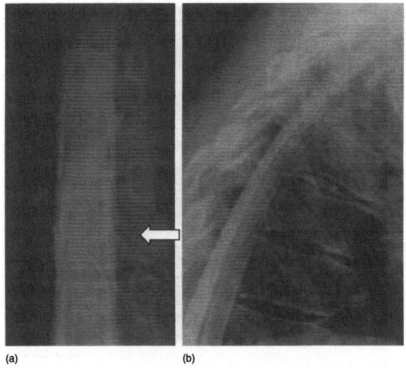

(a)   (b)

Fig. 33.2 Myelogram showing leakage of contrast into the subdural space (arrow).

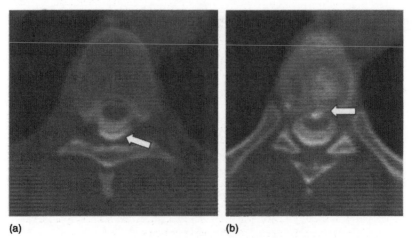

(a)   (b)

Fig. 33.3 CT spine performed 20 minutes post-myelogram showing subdural enhancement where the contrast has leaked out into the subdural space (arrow). The right-hand image shows a calcified thoracic disc and calcified disc material impinging on the cord possibly the cause of the CSF leak.

contrast from a dural tear. MRI changes show meningeal thickening with gadolinium enhancement, subdural fluid collection, and evidence of brain descent (cerebellar tonsillar descent resembling Chiari type I, diminution of the prepontine, perichiasmiatic and subarachnoid cisterns, inferior displacement of the optic chiasm, and descent of the iter, the opening of the aqueduct of Sylvius as seen on midsaggital MRI). Identification of the site of the CSF leak usually requires spinal imaging using myelography and CT. Dural tears identified in this way may be treated surgically.

LP produces dry taps in 50%, the majority of patients have pressure less than 6cm but only 50% have pressures lower than 4cm. Pleocytosis of CSF is common (up to 40 mononuclear cells/mm^3) and the protein concentration may be modestly increased.

33d) The most effective treatment of spontaneous intracranial hypotension is unclear since there are no data from large randomized trials.

Treatments currently in use include bedrest and hydration, steroids, caffeine, epidural saline injection, and application of an autologous lumbar epidural blood patch, in which 10–20ml of the patient's own blood is injected into the epidural space at the site of presumed CSF leakage. This patient received an autologous blood patch with good results. Injecting blood into the epidural space carries a small risk of inducing cauda equina compression, infection or SAH, but these complications are unlikely if the blood volume is small and injected gently. Surgery has been performed on a few patients including ligation of meningeal diverticulae and epidural space packing for focal CSF leaks and has been reported to relieve headache within 24 hours. However, the indications for surgery are not established at present.

Further reading

Grimaldi D, Mea E, Chiapparini L, et al (2004). Spontaneous low cerebrospinal pressure: a mini review. Neurol Sci; 25 Suppl 3:S135–137. Review.

Mokri B, Piepgras DG, Miller GM (1997). Syndrome of orthostatic headaches and diffuse pachymeningeal gadolinium enhancement. May Clin Proc; 72:400–413.

Renowden SA, Gregory R, Hyman N, Hilton-Jones D (1995). Spontaneous intracranial hypotension. J Neurol Neurosurg Psychiatry; 59(5):511–515.

Schievink WI, Morreale VM, Atkinson JL et al (1998). Surgical treatment of spontaneous spinal cerebrospinal fluid leaks. J Neurosurg; 88:243–246.

Spelle L, Boulin A, Pierot L, Graveleau P, Tainturier C (1997). Spontaneous intracranial hypotension: MRI and radionuclidcisternography findings. JNNP; 62(3):291–292.

Case 34

A 30-year-old woman was admitted with sudden onset headache, vomiting, dizziness and photophobia. The only past medical history of note was of recurrent migraine with aura 10 years previously. On examination, she was alert with a temperature of 37.8°C, neck stiffness and photophobia but no focal neurology. Intravenous ceftriaxone was given. Five hours later, her GCS had dropped to 10 and she developed a right hemiparesis.

Investigations showed:

- WCC 12×10^9/L, CRP 40mg/L
- U&E and glucose normal, thyroid autoantibodies negative
- CT brain with contrast: normal
- LP: clear fluid, opening pressure 13cm H_2O, no xanthochromia or cells, normal protein and glucose.

She was transferred to intensive care where, over the next few hours, she developed a swinging fever, GCS remained reduced at 9 and there was a variable right-sided weakness that evolved into a dense right hemiparesis. MR imaging of brain and vessels was normal. The following day, there was a slight improvement but she remained pyrexial with right-sided weakness. Repeat MRI and CSF were normal. EEG showed bitemporal slowing.

Questions

34a) Give the differential diagnosis that you would have considered prior to the investigation results.

34b) What is the most likely diagnosis in the light of the investigation results, and why?

34c) What further investigations would you request?

34d) What is the prognosis?

Answers

34a) The differential diagnosis is for an encephalopathy with focal neurological abnormality preceded by headache and is wide including:

- Vascular disorders
  - SAH/intracerebral haemorrhage
  - CVT
  - Cerebral arterial dissection
  - Cerebral vasculitis
  - Call-Fleming syndrome.
- Infection
  - Meningitis/encephalitis/cerebral abscess.
- Neoplastic disorder
- Other
  - Migraine
  - CADASIL
  - MELAS
  - Hashimoto's encephalopathy
  - Drugs e.g. cocaine.

SAH should always be considered in a patient with sudden onset headache and in this case there were additional features (photophobia, depressed conscious level, neck stiffness and focal neurological signs) consistent with this diagnosis. **Meningitis or encephalitis** may cause similar symptoms and signs but the headache is not usually sudden in onset. Headache occurs in the majority (75%) of cases of **CVT** (see page 10) and there may be depressed conscious level and focal neurological signs that can fluctuate. This patient did not appear to have any risk factors for CVT but this does not exclude the diagnosis. **Cerebral arterial dissection** (see page 118) frequently causes head or facial pain that may be acute in onset and may cause focal neurological signs if there is associated thrombosis. However, one would not expect such a rapid decline in conscious level in the absence of brainstem signs indicating brainstem infarction unless there was associated SAH, which occurs rarely in cranial arterial dissection (almost always in the posterior circulation). **Cerebral vasculitis** (see page 174) and the syndrome of metabolic encephalopathy, lactic acidosis and stroke-like episodes (**MELAS**) (see page 103) cause reduced conscious level and focal neurological changes but one would not expect a sudden onset severe headache in either of these conditions. Likewise, cerebral autosomal dominant angiopathy with subcortical infarcts and leucoencephalopathy (**CADASIL**) (see page 71), although associated with migraine and strokes would not be expected to produce an acute encephalopathy.

Migraine coma with hemiplegia (see below) would be a likely diagnosis particularly in view of the history of migraine. **Reversible cerebral vasoconstriction** is seen in migraine (and 'migraine variants' such as thunderclap headache) and is a possible mechanism for the prolonged neurological deficits and strokes associated with this disorder. The **Call–Fleming syndrome** (or posterior cerebral vascoconstriction syndrome) which is also associated with reversible cerebral vasoconstriction, is a rare disorder that typically presents dramatically with sudden onset headache, nausea, vomiting, seizures and focal neurological deficits (often localized to the occipital lobes) and patients are often assumed to have SAH. It is usually seen in pregnancy or the puerperium but may occur spontaneously. Since the Call–Fleming syndrome and thunderclap headache are frequently associated with migraine, the distinction between the Call–Fleming syndrome and migraine-associated vasospasm is not clear. Pre-eclampsia/eclampsia should be considered in pregnant women with headache, encephalopathy, photophobia and visual abnormalities. **Hypertensive encephalopathy** is rarely seen nowadays, but should be considered in hypertensive patients with headache and reduced conscious level. **Hashimoto's encephalopathy** (see page 98) causes stroke-like episodes and encephalopathy but the CSF protein is usually elevated.

34b) Further investigation includes:

- Blood and CSF lactate (to exclude MELAS)
- Cerebral angiography.

Cerebral angiography might be considered if cerebral vasculitis, CVT or Call–Fleming syndrome were thought to be the underlying cause but should probably avoided in this case where migraine is the most likely diagnosis because of the danger of precipitating vasospasm.

34c) The most likely diagnosis is **migraine coma with hemiplegia** (familial hemiplegic migraine).

The diagnosis of migraine coma with hemiplegia is essentially one of exclusion. The clinical features of this case could be consistent with **SAH or CNS infection** but the normal CT brain with absence of xanthochromia in the CSF rules out SAH and normal CSF makes

CNS infection very unlikely. **CVT** can present with sudden-onset headache and the normal MR imaging of the brain and cerebral vessels does not exclude CVT but the presence of persistent focal neurological signs in absence of any evidence of venous infarction on MRI would be atypical. **Arterial dissection** is not excluded by a normal magnetic resonance angiogram since the resolution of this technique is not sufficient to visualize all dissections (see page 115). However, the clinical features are not consistent with this diagnosis since one would again expect brain imaging findings consistent with a stroke. **Cerebral vasculitis** is not excluded by a normal MRI/MRA and CSF but is unlikely in view of the clinical history of sudden onset headache in someone previously well. The only likely diagnoses that would explain the clinical picture and the investigation results are **migraine** (and the rare Call–Fleming syndrome). The past history of migraine with aura is consistent with this diagnosis.

Migraine coma with hemiplegia (or familial hemiplegic migraine) was described in the 19th century by Charcot, Osler, and Gowers, amongst others. There is recurrent coma and hemiplegia which often alternate and may be precipitated by exercise and minor trauma. Initial presentation is usually in childhood or early adulthood. Attacks are characterized by headache, fever, meningism and fluctuating conscious level with a leucocytosis often resulting in a diagnosis of meningoencephalitis. Focal neurological signs may be present including episodic or progressive ataxia. Imaging is usually normal and there may be a CSF pleocytosis. EEG typically shows temporal slow waves. Angiography should be avoided because of the risk of precipitating vasospasm.

Migraine coma with hemiplegia is usually a familial condition associated with a mutation in the calcium channel α1 subunit gene, CACNA1A gene, located on chromosome 19p13. Mutations in the same gene have also been found in some hereditary ataxias including episodic ataxia and some of the spinocerebellar ataxias indicating that these disorders and migraine coma with hemiplegia are channelopathies. Recently, a new locus for migraine coma with hemiplegia has been found on chromosome 1 in a region reported to contain another calcium channel subunit gene. Sporadic cases also occur in which similar genetic abnormalities may be found. The mechanism by which reversible neurological deficit and coma occur is not known but it is thought that there may be a metabolic abnormality leading to transient neuronal dysfunction.

34d) The prognosis for migraine coma with hemiplegia is generally good. Resolution of symptoms within 2–7 days usually occurs but deaths have been reported. This patient made a complete recovery.

Further reading

Ducros A, Tournier-Lasserve E, Bousser MG (2002). The genetics of migraine. *Lancet Neurol;* 1(5):285–293. Review.

Ducros A, Denier C, Joutel A, Cecillon M, Lescoat C, Vahedi K, Darcel F, Vicant E, Bousser MG, Tournier-Lasserve E (2001). The clinical spectrum of familial hemiplegic migraine associated with mutations in a neuronal calcium channel. *N Engl J Med;* 345(1):17–24.

Koeppen AH (2003). Familial hemiplegic migraine. *Arch Neurol;* 60(5):663–664. Review

Case 35

A 38-year-old male car mechanic presented with a 2-month history of poor coordination, memory impairment and urinary incontinence. Over the previous year he had also become more withdrawn with reduced appetite and some weight loss and there had been uncharacteristic absences from work. His family doctor had diagnosed depression 3 months previously and treated him with an antidepressant. There was no significant past medical history or family history. He drank a moderate amount of alcohol and denied smoking or taking illegal drugs.

On examination there was a global reduction in cognitive function but speech was preserved, although with confabulation. There was poor initiation of tasks and a calm affect. There were no involuntary movements, tone was increased but power and sensation were preserved. The reflexes were brisk bilaterally and the plantars extensor. The gait was ataxic. Fundi, eye movements and the rest of the cranial nerves were normal.

Investigations showed:

- MRI (see Fig. 35.1)
- EEG: diffuse slow wave abnormalities
- CSF: normal.

Questions

35a) Give a differential diagnosis.

35b) What does the arrow indicate on the MRI?

35c) What is the most likely diagnosis?

35d) What other diagnostic investigations would you request, if any? What are the drawbacks of these investigations?

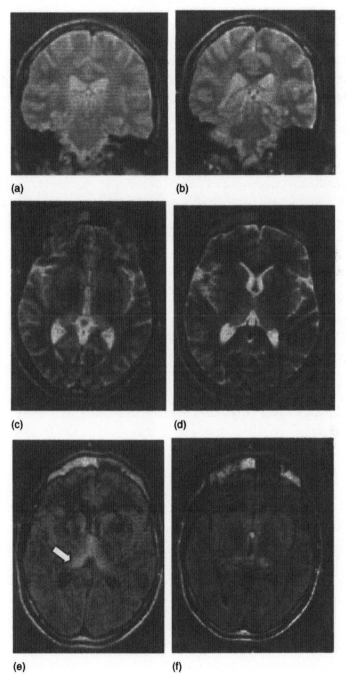

(a)

(b)

(c)

(d)

(e)

(f)

Fig. 35.1

Answers

35a) The clinical features of this case indicate an encephalopathy with ataxia on a background of personality change and the initial differential diagnosis is wide:

- Infection:
  - HIV (see pages 87 and 263)
  - Atypical agents including cryptococcus (see page 42), toxoplasma
  - TB (see page 54).
- Degenerative disease:
  - New variant CJD (nvCJD)
  - Huntington's disease
  - Spinocerebellar atrophy.
- Inflammatory conditions:
  - MS
  - Vasculitis (see page 174)
  - Hashimoto's encephalitis (see page 98).
- Vascular disorders:
  - CADASIL (see page 71).
- Structural lesion:
  - Space-occupying lesions
  - Hydrocephalus.
- Toxic/metabolic disorders:
  - Wilson's disease (see page 218)
  - Hypothyroidism [usually peripheral neuropathy/myopathy (see page 35)]
  - B12 deficiency [usually peripheral neuropathy (see page 268)]
  - Alcohol (see page 18)
  - Mercury poisoning (see page 49)
  - Vitamin E deficiency (see page 48)
  - Pellagra (see page 49).
- Neoplasia:
  - Multiple metastases
  - Paraneoplastic disorders (see page 252).

35b) The MRI shown in Fig. 35.1 shows coronal proton density (upper row), axial T2-weighted (middle row) and axial FLAIR (lower row) images. The arrow indicates an area of **high signal in the pulvinar**, a large nucleus in the most posterior part of the thalamus that has extensive connections with parietal, temporal and occipital association cortices.

35c) The most likely diagnosis is **nvCJD**.

The clinical features together with the imaging findings are consistent with nvCJD. The median age of nv CJD sufferers is 29 years (range 18–53 years) and the median illness duration prior to death is 14 months (range 8–38 months). There is early psychiatric disturbance in all patients and ataxia develops after approximately 6 months. Chorea and dystonia often appear before myoclonus. Bilateral pulvinar high signal is sensitive (around 78%) and specific (around 100%) for nvCJD.

The diagnostic criteria for new variant CJD are as follows:

- I
  - progressive neuropsychiatric disorder
  - illness duration > 6 months
  - routine investigation does not suggest another diagnosis
  - no history of potential iatrogenic exposure
- II
  - early psychiatric symptoms
  - persistent painful sensory symptoms
  - ataxia
  - myoclonus, chorea, dystonia
  - dementia
- IIIA
  - EEG not suggestive of sporadic CJD
- IIIB
  - bilateral pulvinar high signal on MRI

The EEG in nv CJD does not show the classic tri-phasic complexes seen in the sporadic form. Usually there is non-specific slow wave activity but the EEG can be normal. The diagnosis of nvCJD is 'definite' if there is a progressive neuropsychiatric disorder and neuropathological confirmation; 'probable' if there is all of I and 4 out of 5 of II and IIIA + IIIB; and 'possible' if there is all of I and 4 out of 5 of II and IIIA.

35d) Further investigations include:

- 14–3–3 protein assay
- tonsillar biopsy.

CSF immunoassay for protein 14–3–3 may be performed (protein 14–3–3 reflects extensive destruction of brain tissue) but this protein may be elevated in other conditions associated with brain damage including recent stroke, meningoencephalitis and cerebral intravascular lymphoma. Nevertheless, one study reported 97% sensitivity and 87% specificity for nvCJD. Tonsillar biopsy has been performed in a few patients with nvCJD and in one study all 8 patients had abnormal prion protein present in tonsillar samples. The prion protein genotype differs from that of other forms of CJD.

Further reading

Green AJ, Thompson EJ, Stewart GE *et al* (2001). Use of 14-3-3 and other brain-specific proteins in CSF in the diagnosis of variant Creutzfeldt-Jakob disease. *J Neurol Neurosurg Psychiatry;* **70**(6):744–748.

Hill AF, Butterworth RJ, Joiner S *et al* (1999). Investigation of variant Creutzfelt–Jakob disease and other prion diseases with tonsil biopsy samples. *Lancet;* **353**(9148): 183–189.

Malluci G, Collinge J (2004). Update on Creutzfeldt–Jakob disease. *Curr Opin Neurol;* **17**(6):641–647.

Zeidler M, Sellar RJ, Collie DA *et al* (2000). The pulvinar sign on magnetic resonance imaging in variant Creutzfeldt–Jakob disease. *Lancet;* **355**:1412-1418.

Case 36

A 20-year-old male student presented to the emergency department having awoken with slurred speech, difficulty swallowing solids, and problems walking. He had also noticed intermittent involuntary movement of his thumbs across his palms over the past few weeks together with occasional indistinct speech. There was no past medical or family history of note although he had lost weight over the preceeding year and a decline in his rugby skills had been noted by his team-mates. He denied drug use and was on no medication.

On examination he looked well and general systems were normal. He had dysarthria, slow tongue movements and a brisk jaw jerk. There was increased tone in the limbs with intermittent dystonic posturing of the arms. Reflexes were normal. His gait was ataxic.

Investigations

Routine blood tests including FBC, reticulocyte count, clotting, TFT and inflammatory markers were unremarkable apart from a mildly raised GGT at 60IU/L. CT and MRI brain (see Fig. 36.1) were performed.

Questions

36a) Give a differential diagnosis.

36b) What is the most likely diagnosis?

36c) What investigations would you perform to provide further evidence for this diagnosis?

36d) Is there a diagnostic test?

36e) Describe the MRI abnormalities in this patient. What are the typical neuroradiological findings of this condition?

36f) Describe the various ways in which this condition may present.

36g) How would you manage this patient?

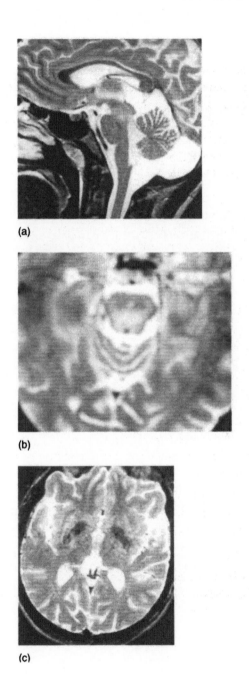

(a)

(b)

(c)

Fig. 36.1

Answers

36a) This patient presents with a movement disorder, dysarthria, ataxia and dystonia. The differential diagnosis includes:

- Vascular disease:
  - Stroke, vasculitis.
- Metabolic disease:
  - Wilson's disease
  - Hypocalcaemia
  - Hyperglycaemia (hemiballism/hemichorea), hypoglycaemia
  - Hyper/hyponatraemia, hypomagnesaemia.
- Endocrine disease:
  - Thyroid disease (usually chorea in hypertyroidism and ataxia in hypothyroidism).
- Perinatal hypoxia (latency may be up to 58 years)
- Toxins:
  - Carbon monoxide
  - Cyanide
  - Methanol
  - Mercury (see page 49).
- Drugs:
  - Metoclopramide
  - Anticonvulsants
  - Dopamine agonists
  - Neuoleptics.
- Infection:
  - Sydenham's chorea associated with rheumatic fever (group A strep-toccocal infection).
  - Mycoplasma pneumoniae
  - Legionella
  - Varicella (children)
  - HIV
  - Toxoplasma.
- Inflammatory disease:
  - e.g. SLE/antiphospholipid syndrome (chorea usually)

- Polyarteritis nodosa
- Behçet's.
- Paraneoplastic syndrome:
  - e.g. oat cell carcinoma with anti-Hu antibody (see page 252).
- Space-occupying lesion:
  - e.g. of brain stem causing tongue dystonia.
- Inherited conditions:
  - Huntington's disease
  - Spinocerebellar ataxia.

36b) The most likely diagnosis is **Wilson's disease.**

The most likely diagnosis is Wilson's disease since the history and examination do not suggest any of the alternative causes. This is supported by the radiological abnormalities. Wilson's disease is an inherited autosomal recessive disorder of copper accumulation caused by impaired copper excretion into the bile. It must be considered in any young or middle-aged person presenting with a movement disorder, dysarthria, or personality change. Onset of symptoms is unusual before the age of 6 years or after the age of 40 years, although presentations as late as 60-years-old have been recorded.

36c) Further investigation should include:

- Slit lamp examination to look for Kayser–Fleischer rings (copper deposits around the margin of the cornea in Descemet's membrane) (see below)
- 24-hour urinary copper (usually increased) and serum caeruloplasmin (usually decreased)
- Liver ultrasound looking for cirrhosis.

Kayser–Fleischer rings are suggestive but not diagnostic of Wilson's disease (they may also occur in severe cholestatic liver disease). They are present in all patients with neurological symptoms. In this patient, caeruloplasmin was 3mg/dL (normal ≤16mg/dL) and urinary copper was 83μmol/24 hours (normal ≤0.9μmol/24 hours). It should be noted that both urinary copper and serum caeruloplasmin may be within the normal range. Liver ultrasound suggested cirrhotic changes but no portal hypertension. Most patients presenting with neurological symptoms are cirrhotic but synthetic liver function and transaminase levels may be normal.

36d) The tests listed in 36c are not diagnostic and DNA analysis should be requested.

None of the abnormalities described in 36c is specific to Wilson's disease and thus is not diagnostic of the disorder. DNA analysis shows a mutation in *ATP7B* (Wilson) gene on chromosome 13 as was seen in this patient. The Wilson's gene encodes a copper binding ATP-ase. There are over 200 mutations in the Wilson's gene described so far. It has been suggested that the different mutations are responsible for the wide phenotypic variation seen in Wilson's disease but at present there is little evidence for clear phenotype-genotype correlation.

36e) The T2–weighted MRI brain shows hyperintensity in the midbrain, caudate and putamen and hypointensity in the pallidum.

Brain imaging in Wilson's disease may be normal, particularly in patients with mild or asymptomatic disease. CT may show low signal in the basal ganglia and MRI abnormalities include signal change and rarely lytic lesions, in the basal ganglia and midbrain as seen in this patient (see also Fig. 36.2 showing more extensive MRI abnormalities in a severely affected patient). In advanced cases, there is cortical atrophy and ventricular dilatation. Therapy may improve the appearance of the basal ganglia lesions.

36f) Approximately one-third of patients with Wilson's disease present with liver disease, one third with neurological symptoms, and one-third with psychiatric features.

Children usually present with an acute jaundice caused by haemolysis in the presence of cirrhosis or chronic hepatitis which may be rapidly fatal. Systemic manifestations include anorexia, nausea, weight loss, splenomegaly and easy bruising.

The mean age for onset of neurological symptoms is 21 years. The major neurological symptoms are dysarthria and drooling, poor coordination, tremor, dystonia, bradykinesia, rigidity, and gait abnormality. Psychiatric changes are usually insidious and include personality change, intellectual decline, depression, and emotional lability.

36g) Early diagnosis and treatment are of paramount importance if further deterioration is to be prevented.

First line treatment is with penicillamine with pyridoxine supplementation. Half of patients with established disease show initial improvement on therapy, 15% remain stable, and the remainder deteriorate. Initial deterioration in symptoms may be minimised by gradually increasing

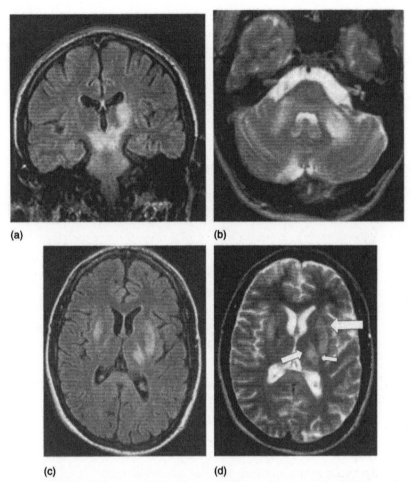

(a)

(b)

(c)

(d)

Fig. 36.2 MRI brain from a patient with severe Wilson's disease showing hyperintensity in the midbrain and left lateral thalamus (coronal T1-weighted image, a), diffuse high signal in both cerebellar peduncles (axial T2-weighted image, b), and hyperintensity in the left internal capsule, lateral thalamus and putamen (small, medium and large arrows respectively) on T1-weighted (c) and T2-weighted (d) axial slices.

the penicillamine dose. Side effects of penicillamine are many and include rash, lupus like syndrome, myasthaenia like syndrome, and glomerulonephritis. Alternative treatment is with trientene or zinc if neither the latter nor penicillamine is tolerated. Zinc competes for copper absorption in the intestine and stimulates metallothione (metallobinding protein) production in the liver which binds copper.

Treatment of Wilson's disease should be lifelong and patients should be warned that sudden discontinuation of therapy causes rapid acute deterioration.

Further reading

Brewer GJ, Fink JK, Hedera P (1999). Diagnosis and treatment of Wilson's disease. *Semin Neurol*; 19(3):261–277.

Ferenci P (2004). Pathophysiology and clinical features of Wilson disease. *Metab Brain Dis*; 19(3–4):229–239.

Jones EA, Weissenborn K (1997). Neurology and the liver. *J Neurol Neurosurg Psychiatry*; 63(3):279–293.

Robertson WM (2000). Wilson's disease. *Arch Neurol*; 57(2):276–277.

Case 37

A 40-year-old man had a 6-week history of headache that had come on gradually over the frontal area and then become generalized. It was worst on waking and coughing, and there was some relief from paracetamol and diclofenac. Over the last 3 days he had double vision in all directions of vision, except to the right. On examination, he was slim, normotensive and afebrile. There was decreased visual acuity of 6/9 on the left and double vision except on looking to the right. There was bilateral papilloedema. Blood tests including inflammatory markers were normal. He had a normal CT scan, MRI/MRV and CSF.

Questions

37a) What is the diagnosis, and why does he have double vision?

37b) What is unusual about this case?

37c) What other diagnosis may mimic this condition?

37d) What investigation would confirm your diagnosis?

37e) How would you treat this patient and how would you monitor his condition?

Answers

37a) The diagnosis is **idiopathic (benign) intracranial hypertension (IIH)**.

Diagnosis of IIH depends on the exclusion of other causes of raised intracranial pressure. IIH presents with headache that is diffuse, worse at night or on waking in the morning, may cause nocturnal waking and be excacerbated by coughing. Transient obscuration of vision can occur with sudden change in position. Double vision from VI nerve palsy is often associated with IIH as the nerve is stretched by shifts in cerebral tissue. Other symptoms include ataxia and paraesthesia, but objective signs on examination are rare. Seizures may occur, but are rare and should lead to considertion of alternative diagnoses. Examination reveals papilloedema and possibly an enlarged blind spot.

37b) This case is atypical in that the patient is a slim male.

Patients with IIH are usually overweight, young-to-middle-aged females, often with menstrual irregularities. There is some evidence that males with IIH do not tend to be overweight in contrast to women with IIH, but it is often difficult to be certain in individual cases that the syndrome of IIH is not due to recent **CVT** which is no longer evident on imaging (see below). Further, the diagnosis of IIH should always be reconsidered if it is resistant to treatment or if other symptoms develop (see Fig. 37.1).

37c) **CVT** may mimic IIH.

A significant proportion of patients diagnosed as having IIH, probably at least 25%, have CVT (see page 10). Patients diagnosed with IIH who are subsequently found to have CVT, are often male, and of normal build. It could be argued that MRV should be performed in all cases of IIH particularly when the clinical features are atypical. Conditions previously thought to cause IIH including otitis media, OCP, pregnancy and various haematological disorders are associated with CVT and thus secondary intracranial hypertension.

The cause of true IIH is unknown. Endocrine abnormalities have not been found despite the higher prevalence in overweight females and the association with polycystic ovarian syndrome. Drugs associated with IIH include tetracycline-type antibiotics, sulphonamides, prednisolone and nitrofurantoin. Recently, venous sinus stenosis has been found to be present in some patients.

37d) Measurement of CSF opening pressure and examination of CSF.

The CSF shows elevated opening pressure (31cm H_2O in the current patient) with normal constituents. Measurement of CSF pressure should

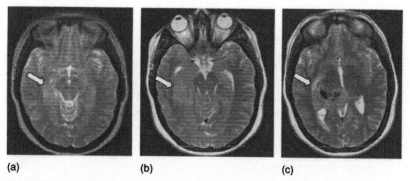

(a)   (b)   (c)

Fig. 37.1 T2-weighted MRI showing an ependymoma of the right temporal lobe (b and c) in a patient thought to have IIH. On close inspection, the tumour can be seen on the initial scan (a) performed a couple of years earlier.

be performed with legs extended and the spine unflexed, particularly in obese patients in whom pressures of 20–30cm H_2O are otherwise commonly found. It should be noted that CSF pressure does vary from time to time in patients with IIH and so a single normal pressure does not exclude the diagnosis if the clinical context is suggestive.

37e) Treatment of IIH involves:

- LP to drain CSF
- Diuretics
- Shunt insertion.

Intracranial pressure should be reduced to relieve symptoms and avoid visual loss. Removal of CSF is the first–line treatment and repeated LPs may be necessary. The most effective long-term treatment in the overweight patient with IIH is weight loss. Drug treatments include acetazolamide, an inhibitor of carbonic anhydrase that lowers CSF production, and furosemide. Steroids have been used but intracranial pressure may increase as they are tapered.

Patients' vision should be monitored carefully with visual field and blind spot measurement, and a fundus camera to monitor the extent of papilloedema. In severe cases, when the papilloedema spreads into the macula, visual acuity falls steeply and blindness may occur. If LP and drugs fail to lower intracranial pressure and vision is threatened, lumboperitoneal shunting may be considered, although shunt malfunction is common. Fenestration of the optic nerve sheath to allow drainage into the orbit is an alternative method of protecting vision.

Further reading

Friedman DI, Jacobsen DM (2002). Diagnostic criteria for idiopathic intracranial hypertension. *Neurology;* **59**:1492–1495.

Kesler A, Goldhammer Y, Gadoth N (2001). Do men with pseudomotor cerebri share the same characteristics as women? A retrospective review of 141 cases. *J Neuroopthalmol;* **21**(3):235.

Ramadan NM (1996). Headache caused by raised intracranial pressure and intracranial hypotension. Curr *Opinions Neurol;* **9**(3): 214–218.

Case 38

A 30-year-old woman had received a renal transplant 4 years previously following renal failure secondary to IgA nephropathy. Ten days prior to admission, she developed an occipital headache worse on movement and coughing. This was followed 3 days later by malaise, shivers, and nocturnal sweats. Three days prior to admission, she became emotionally labile and then dysarthric. She was taking prednisolone 5mg, ciclosporin 1g bd, mycophenolate 150mg bd, nifedipine and ranitidine. Recent investigations by the renal clinic had shown no evidence of graft rejection, a glomerular filtration rate of 50 ml/min, and normal ciclosporin levels.

On examination, she was tearful with a profound scanning dysarthria. Eye movements were full but there were broken saccades, poor pursuit on looking to the right and impersistence of right and vertical gaze. Tongue movements were slow. There was mild right upper limb dysmetria and brisk reflexes. Lower limbs had normal tone and power with brisk knee jerks but absent ankle jerks and plantar reflexes were downgoing. Joint position sense was preserved but there was bilateral loss of pain and temperature to the knees. Heel shin test was normal. Romberg's test was negative. There was mild truncal ataxia, with a tendency to veer to the right. General systems were unremarkable.

Investigations showed:

- Hb 13.3g/dL, WCC 7.3 × 10^9/L, (neutrophils 52%, lymphocytes 21%, monocytes 9%)
- Urea 10.8 mmo/L, Cr 246 μmol/L, LFT normal
- CRP<8 g/dL, ESR 7mm/h
- Cyclosporin level within therapeutic limits
- CXR and CT brain normal
- CSF: opening pressure 18cm H$_2$O, 100 cells/mm^3 (82 lymphocytes, 18 polymorphs), glucose 3.4mm/L (blood glucose 6.2mm/L), protein 0.52 g/L.

Questions

38a) What are the neurological syndromes commonly seen in patients who have undergone renal transplantation?

38b) Describe the anatomical abnormalities underlying the neurological signs in this case.

38c) Give a differential diagnosis.

38d) What further investigations would you perform?

38e) List the neurological complications of ciclosporin therapy.

Answers

38a) Post transplant neurological syndromes include:

- Alteration in mood or frank psychosis secondary to steroids.
- Seizures:
  - Hypertension
  - Cyclosporin
  - Space occupying lesion caused by infection
  - Metabolic derangement e.g. low Mg associated with cyclosporin
  - Rejection encephalopathy.
- Tremor secondary to cyclosporin.
- Peripheral neuropathy:
  - Uraemia
  - Cyclosporin
  - Secondary to the underlying condition causing renal failure eg diabetes mellitus.
- Myopathy:
  - Steroids
  - Statin therapy.
- Inflammatory/infective conditions (see below).

38b) The clinical features of this case suggest:

- Right pontine lesion (see Fig. 38.1)
- Small fibre peripheral neuropathy.

Scanning dysarthria, truncal ataxia (cerebellar vermis) to the right and the right upper limb dysmetria (cerebellar hemisphere) suggest a lesion affecting the cerebellum or the pontocerebellar connections. Damage to the paramedian pontine reticular formation results in an inability to look towards the side of the lesion. There does not appear to be a centre for vertical gaze but lesions in the dorsal brainstem are known to affect upgaze (Parinaud's syndrome). Pursuit movements in which the eyes lock onto a visual target are controlled by visual input to cortical area 19 which projects to the midbrain and pons. Emotional lability together with slow tongue movements occur in pseudobulbar palsy in which descending cortical control of the brainstem motor nuclei is interrupted. Brisk limb jerks might be expected in an upper motor neuron lesion although limb tone and plantar reflexes were normal.

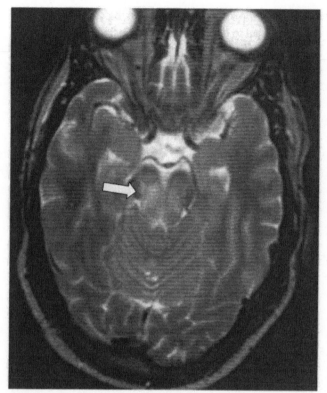

Fig. 38.1 Axial T2-weighted MRI from this patient showing hyperintensity in the right pons (arrow).

The ankle jerks were absent and there was a loss of pain and temperature sensation bilaterally consistent with a small fibre peripheral neuropathy.

38c) The differential diagnosis (most likely diagnoses this far out from transplant shown in italics) includes:

- Opportunistic infection:
  - Viral (*CMV*, VZV, HSV)
  - Bacterial (*listeria*, nocardia, TB)
  - Fungal (*cryptococcus*, aspergillus)
  - Parasitic (toxoplasma).
- Neoplasm (lymphoma).
- Vasculitis.

The peripheral neuropathy in this patient is more likely to be caused by previous uraemia (neuropathy occurs in 60% of patients who reach dialysis), cyclosporin, or to the underlying cause for the renal failure, than to be related to the cause of the brainstem lesion.

Opportunistic infection should be high on the list of differential diagnoses in this man who was immunosuppressed. Neurological infections occur in 5–15% of all transplant recipients and are particularly important because about half of the CNS infections that occur in immunocompromised patients result in death. The number of reported agents is enormous but around three-quarters of cases are caused by *Listeria monocytogenes* (the most common cause of post transplant meningitis), *Cryptococcus neoformans* or *Aspergillus fumigatus*. The most important risk factors for the development of an opportunistic infection are the magnitude and length of time of immunosuppression.

Opportunistic agents may cause a variety of CNS syndromes with or without raised intracranial pressure, seizures or stroke-like presentation:

- Acute meningitis:
  - with brainstem signs and /or lower cranial nerve palsies e.g. listeria.
- Subacute meningitis:
  - often with brainstem signs and/or cranial nerve palsies e.g. TB (see page 54), Cryptococcus (see page 42).
- Meningoencephalitis e.g. cryptococcus, toxoplasma (see Fig. 38.2).
- Encephalitis:
  - e.g. HSV (see page 4), VZV, CMV.

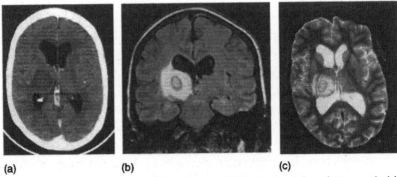

(a) (b) (c)

Fig. 38.2 CT (a) and MRI (coronal FLAIR and axial T2-weighted, b and c respectively) from a patient with toxoplasmosis. Note the intense flare around the central mass lesion indicating extensive surrounding oedema.

- Progressive dementia:
  - e.g. progressive multifocal leucoencephalopathy (PML) caused by the JC virus (see page 87), measles.
- Space occupying lesion:
  - e.g. TB, fungi, nocardia, toxoplasma.

The predominant lymphocyte subgroup on CSF examination varies according to the infecting organism: B cells are predominant in meningitis or abscess, encapsulated organisms (streptococcus, staphylococcus), and pseudomonas, whereas T-cells are raised with intracellular organisms, viruses and fungi, listeria, nocardia, and parasites. Involvement of sites outside the CNS may provide clues: lung involvement occurs in listeria, TB, aspergillus, cryptococcus, and CMV, skin involvement occurs in cryptococcus and gastrointestinal, and retinal involvement is seen in CMV.

Another clue to the causative organism is the time period after transplantation. Up to one month post transplant, infections are rare. Infections occurring in this period will often have been present pretransplant, acquired from the donor or related to indwelling catheters or the surgical procedure itself. Between 1 and 6 months is the peak period for opportunistic infection. Viruses, especially CMV and EBV infection, themselves cause immunosuppression and predispose to listeria, nocardia, candida, and aspergillus. Six months or later after transplant, patients may have lingering viral infection e.g. progressive CMV retinitis or EBV associated lymphoma, or PML, cryptococcus, nocardia, listeria, or infections similar to those found in non immunosupressed populations. Opportunistic infections in the late phase are commonest in patients with chronic graft rejection requiring high doses of immunosuppressants.

The presence of fevers and night sweats in this case is suggestive of **TB** (although one would usually expect a higher CSF protein in TB) but might also indicate **lymphoma**. TB may reactivate post transplantation and high-risk patients are often given prophylactic isoniazid. CNS TB may present as a space-occupying lesion (tuberculoma) or as a basal meningitis (see page 54), often with associated cranial nerve palsies. Treatment is complicated by the fact that antituberculous medication (in particular rifampicin) interacts with steroids and cyclosporin through induction of the cytochrome p450 system: increased immunosuppressive therapy doses are required to avoid transplant rejection.

Lymphoproliferative syndromes occur after prolonged immuno-suppression and are associated with EBV infection. CNS involvement occurs in 15–25% of patients with post transplant lymphoproliferative disorders and it is the only site of detectable disease in 85% of these individuals. MRI shows lesions with mass effect and gadolinium enhancement.

A **vasculitic process** (see page 176) could cause both CNS and peripheral nerve involvement and is a common underlying cause of renal failure. There are no specific features to suggest **Lyme disease** (see page 92) or **brucellosis,** both of which can cause central and peripheral nervous system abnormalities.

38d) Further investigations include:

- MRI brain with gadolinium
- TB: CSF stain and culture for AFB, PCR of CSF
- Cryptococcus: indian ink stain of CSF and cryptoccal antigen
- Listeria: CSF culture
- Nocardia: prolonged (3 weeks) culture of biopsy or aspirate e.g. of brain abscess
- Aspergillus: CSF culture
- Toxoplasma: serology
- Viral infections: CSF PCR
- Lymphoma: CSF cytology.

38e) Ciclosporin causes neurological side effects in 15–40% of patients including:

- Tremor
- Encephalopathy
- Seizures
- Neuropathy.

Although higher levels of ciclosporin are generally associated with side-effects, there is no correlation between drug levels and a specific abnormality. Tremor and exacerbation of hypertension with hypertensive encephalopathy and seizures may occur. Neuralgia and neuropathy are rare and are usually predominantly sensory. Both demyelinating and axonal neuropathies have been reported. Side-effects usually reverse completely after stopping the drug.

Further reading

Cunha B.A (2001). Central nervous system infections in the compromised host: a diagnostic approach. *Infect Dis Clin North Am;* **15**(2):567–590. Review.

Singh N. and Hussain S (2000). Infections of the central nervous system in transplant recipients. *Transpl Infect Dis;* **2**(3):101–111. Review.

Case 39

A 29-year-old male photographer presented with a 1-week history of dysuria and foul smelling urine followed by a 5-day history of headache of gradual onset associated with fevers. He had generalized muscular aches and nausea. He had had casual sexual contact with a woman, not his usual partner, 2 weeks previously. He drank 10–15 units of alcohol per week, smoked 10 cigarettes per day and took occasional recreational 'ecstasy' but denied intravenous drug use.

On examination, he was pyrexial at 38.6°C and genital examination revealed a clear penile discharge. There was no photophobia or neck stiffness and no abnormal neurological findings.

Investigations showed:

- MRI brain: normal
- LP: opening pressure 22cm H_2O, white cells 186/mm^3 (12 polymorphs, 174 lymphocytes), red cells 22/mm^3, glucose 2.6mm/L, (blood glucose of 6.3mm/L) protein 2.25g/L, no organisms seen, no growth

Questions

39a) Give the differential diagnosis you would have considered prior to the LP result.

39b) What is the most likely diagnosis and what treatment would you give?

39c) How would you confirm the diagnosis?

39d) Describe the other neurological complications of this condition and how are they caused?

39e) What is the prognosis?

Answers

39a) The differential diagnosis includes:

- Sexually transmitted infection causing penile discharge and systemic symptoms of fever, headache, myalgia and nausea including:
  - Herpes simplex type 2 (HSV-2)
  - Syphilis (*Treponema pallidum*)
  - *Neisseria gonorrhoeae*
  - *Chlamydia trachomatis*
  - Rarely *Trichomonas vaginalis, Mycoplasma genitilium, Ureaplasma urealyticum, Bacteroides* spp.
- Sexually transmitted infection with spread to the CNS causing meningitis:
  - HSV-2
  - Syphilis.

The history of casual sexual contact followed by dysuria and penile discharge suggests a sexually transmitted infection. The latter may be accompanied by systemic symptoms including headache, myalgia and fever. Such systemic symptoms are particularly common in HSV-2 may also cause genital infection HSV-1 and **syphilis**, but the time course of syphilitic infection does not fit the clinical features of this case: in primary syphilis, a chancre, and sometimes urethral discharge, appear 10–90 days after contact and are followed by secondary syphilis 4–10 weeks later in which systemic symptoms including fever, myalgia, lymphadenopathy and rash occur. **HIV infection** may also cause fever, myalgia and a variety of neurological syndromes including headache at the time of seroconversion (see case 263) but this occurs 6–8 weeks after exposure. One would also not expect a urethral discharge from HIV infection although there is often co-infection with other pathogens e.g. gonococcus. The possibility of opportunistic CNS infection associated with immunosuppression from undiagnosed established HIV infection should always be considered in high risk individuals with headache and fever but, in this case, the presence of genitourinary symptoms closely associated with headache and inflammatory CSF suggest a primary sexually transmitted infectious cause. HSV, *N. gonorrhoea* and syphilis may cause neurological syndromes including meningitis. Finally, it should be noted that drugs, such as trimethoprim and ibuprofen, used to treat urinary symptoms may cause meningitis.

39b) The diagnosis is HSV-2 **meningitis.**

The presence of an inflammatory CSF with predominance of lymphocytes is consistent with non-bacterial CNS infection. Together with the clinical picture, this suggests a primary genital infection with secondary infection of the CNS (meningitis).

The most likely diagnosis is HSV-2 infection which is a common cause of sexually transmitted infection and may cause a variety of neurological syndromes (see below) including **aseptic meningitis.** Aseptic meningitis is the term given to meningitis such as that caused by viruses, bacteria that do not grow in routine cultures (e.g. *T. pallidum*, mycoplasma, leptospira, rickettsia, borrelia) and drugs (e.g. carbamazepine and ibuprofen). HSV-2 accounts for 0.5–5% of viral meningitis. At the time of the first attack of HSV-2, around 7% of women and 2% of men develop meningitis although many more will have headache and fever in the absence of obvious CNS involvement. Treatment is with intravenous followed by oral antiviral agents (newer agents such as valaciclovir have better oral bioavailability) although it is unclear how much difference such treatment makes to the outcome. HSV-2 is the most common cause of recurrent aseptic meningitis (20% of those who develop meningitis) and there may be no history of genital symptoms. The clinical syndromes associated with HSV-1 and HSV-2 overlap and thus HSV-1 may cause genital infection although typically it causes an encephalitis (see page 4). Syphilis may cause aseptic meningitis in the secondary phase but as stated above, this occurs 4–10 weeks after primary syphilis and thus does not fit the time course of this case. *N. gonorrhoea* is a rare cause of acute bacterial meningitis.

39c) The diagnosis was confirmed on PCR of the CSF which showed HSV-2. PCR testing and viral culture may be performed on urethral, mouth and throat swabs.

39d) HSV-2 is associated with a number of neurological syndromes including:

- Radiculomyelitis
- Meningitis
- Cranial neuropathy
- Transverse myelitis.

Lumbosacral radiculomyelitis is caused by direct virus spread into the spinal cord causing perineal sensory changes, urinary retention and/or leg weakness. If the primary infection is oral, cranial nerves may be affected and facial sensory change or palsy may occur. Meningitis is discussed above. Encephalitis is rare in comparison to HSV-1, which is the commonest cause of sporadic viral encephalitis in the developed world. Transverse myelitis may also occur.

39e) The prognosis from HSV-2 meningitis is good since this is typically a self-limiting illness. The genital infection however, will not be permanently eradicated and may intermittently flare up causing blistering at which time the patient is infectious.

Further reading

Connolly KJ (1990). The acute aseptic meningitis syndrome. *Infect Dis Clin North America;* **4**(4):599–622.

Johnsson MK, Wahren B (2004). Sexually transmitted herpes simplex viruses. *Scand J Infect Dis;* **36**(2):93–101. Review.

Marques AR, Straus SE (2000). Herpes simplex type 2 infections–an update. *Adv Intern Med;* **45**:175–208. Review.

Case 40

A 50-year-old van driver was admitted to hospital via the surgical team with a 10-day history of lower abdominal and lower back pain radiating into the left groin and the left thigh. He had been constipated and had vomited once and was feverish. There were no urinary symptoms. He had no past medical history apart from an olecranon bursitis 2 months previously following a work injury. He was a non-smoker and drank little alcohol. He was on no regular medication. On examination, he was pyrexial at 38.5°C, with tenderness over the lower abdomen but no guarding, and tenderness in the loins and lower back.

Initial investigations showed:

- Hb 13.7g/dL, WCC 22.7 × 10^9/L (neutrophil leukocytosis), plt 305 × 10^9/L
- Albumin 27g/L, alk phos 286IU/L, bilirubin 35μmol/L, ALT 234IU/L
- U&E and clotting normal
- CXR: normal
- AXR: faecal loading.
- Urine dipstick and microscopy: no blood or protein, no cells, no casts.

He was commenced on intravenous broad spectrum antibiotics. The following day he became progressively confused, agitated and disorientated, and then drowsy. On examination, there was no neck stiffness or other evidence of meningism and there were no focal neurological signs. General systems were normal apart from abdominal tenderness.

Further investigations showed:

- CT brain and abdomen/pelvis (see Figs. 40.1 and 40.2).
- CSF: opening pressure 36cm H_2O, 270 white cells/mm³ (220 polymorphs), 30 red cells/mm³, protein 2g/L, glucose 1mmol/L (blood glucose 6mm/L).

Questions

40a) What does the CT brain scan show? What is indicated by the arrows on the pelvic CT scan?

40b) What is the likely cause of the CT abnormality given the CSF results?

40c) What is the unifying diagnosis that would explain the clinical features of this case?

40d) What further investigations would you request to confirm your diagnosis?

40e) How would you treat this patient?

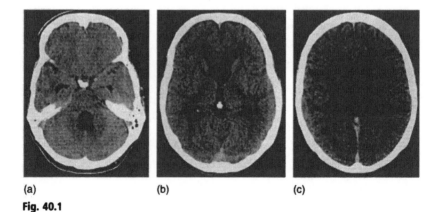

(a)   (b)   (c)

Fig. 40.1

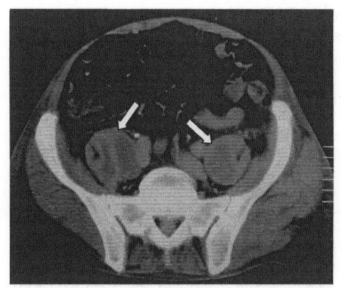

Fig. 40.2

Answers

40a) The CT brain shows **communicating hydrocephalus.** The arrows on the pelvic CT indicate **psoas abscesses.**

There is dilatation of the ventricular system with a reduction in size of the cortical CSF spaces and basal cisterns suggesting raised intracranial pressure. All four ventricles are equally affected consistent with communicating hydrocephalus. There is also loss of cerebral grey/white matter differentiation in keeping with oedema.

40b) **Infective meningitis** is the likely cause of the CT brain abnormality.

The CSF result showing an elevated white cell count with neutrophilia, reduced glucose (normal CSF glucose is around 60% of the blood glucose level), and raised protein, suggests infection. The relatively high protein in the presence of a relatively low cell count could indicate an atypical infection, such as TB (see page 54) (particularly given the high alcohol intake), but is more likely in this case to be due to a bacterial meningitis which has been pre-treated with intravenous antibiotics. The most likely cause of this patient's communicating hydrocephalus is a secondary reduction of CSF resorption through the arachnoid granulations in the dural sinuses secondary to the meningitic infection.

40c) The unifying diagnosis is **olecranon bursitis** leading to *Staphylococcus aureus* septicaemia and **psoas abscess, lumbar discitis, and meningitis.**

The patient presented with back and abdominal pain and was febrile. The initial investigations showed evidence of probable bacterial infection with elevated white cell count and neutrophilia, but the focus of infection was unclear. He subsequently developed confusion and drowsiness, which can occur in association with systemic infection in the elderly, but which would be unexpected in a relatively young patient in the absence of CNS pathology. The clinical findings thus suggested intra-abdominal sepsis with spread to the CNS. CSF was obtained at the time of ventricular drain insertion. The lack of meningism was probably due to the pre-treatment with antibiotics.

Several organisms associated with intra-abdominal infection, including *E. coli, Streptococcus bovis,* Salmonella, *Proteus* species, *Klebsiella* species, and enterobacteriae, may occasionally cause meningitis, particularly in the elderly, patients with chronic medical conditions such as renal or cardiac failure, or following neurosurgical procedures. The cause of the intra-abdominal sepsis in the patient described above was unclear initially. The LFTs were abnormal but not grossly so and there was no tenderness in the hepatic region as would usually but not invariably occur in biliary sepsis or subdiaphragmatic abscess. Abnormal LFTs may occur with systemic sepsis. There were no urinary symptoms and urinary microscopy was unremarkable making pyelonephritis unlikely. Diverticular abscess or colonic cancer would also be unlikely in a man of this age.

The CSF gram stain showed gram-positive cocci consistent with *Staphylococcus aureus* which was confirmed on subsequent culture. Meningitis caused by *Staphylococcus aureus* usually occurs after invasive neurosurgical procedures or after administration of intrathecal therapy. The recent history of olecranon bursitis suggested a possible source of staphylococcal infection in the patient described above. *Staphylococcus aureus* may cause intra-abdominal collections, specifically psoas abscess or subdiaphragmmatic abscess. The location of this man's abdominal pain would be consistent with psoas abscess. Back pain in association with a staphylococcal meningitis, as seen in this patient, should raise the possibility of a discitis and or epidural abscess (see page 168). Discitis and epidural abscess may occur through direct spread of infection from an intra-abdominal source, and is a potential primary source of CNS infection.

40d) Further investigations include:

- Blood, urine, CSF and psoas abcess/discitis aspirate culture
- MRI spine.

Further investigations include blood cultures and urine cultures sent prior to commencement of antibiotics. CT abdomen was performed in this case to look for the source of sepsis and to enable drainage of any intra-abdominal collection. Fluid from the psoas abscesses was sent for microbiological investigation.

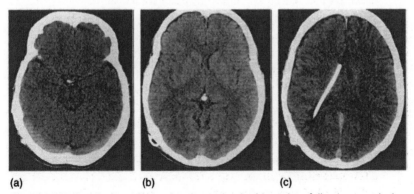

(a) (b) (c)

Fig. 40.3 CT showing ventricular decompression in this patient following ventricular drain insertion (the drain is visible in the right lateral ventricle).

T2-weighted MRI spine showed high signal in the L3/L4 disc with loss of disc height, a small antevertebral fluid collection and an epidural collection over the posterior aspect of L4. There were marrow changes in the vertebral bodies consistent with inflammation. Discs may be aspirated under radiological guidance. Echocardiogram (ideally transoesophageal echocardiography) should be performed to look for valvular vegetations consistent with endocarditis as this may occur following staphylococcal septicaemia (see page 148).

40e) Treatment includes:

- broad spectrum antibiotics
- ventricular drain insertion
- drainage of intra-abdominal collections.

Intravenous broad-spectrum antibiotics with good CNS penetration should be given prior to microbiological diagnosis. The communicating hydrocephalus with associated confusion and drowsiness requires prompt treatment with ventricular drain (see Fig. 40.3) or omaya reservoir insertion. Patients should be observed closely after subsequent drain removal as hydrocephalus may occur. The psoas abcesses should be drained under radiological guidance. Collections of pus associated with a discitis may also be drained in a similar manner.

Further reading

Lee YT, Lee CM, Su SC, Liu CP, Wang TE (1999). Psoas abscess: a 10 year review. *J Microbiol Immunol Infect*; **32**(1):40–46.

Mallick M, Thoufeeq MH, Rajendran TP (2004). Iliopsoas abscesses. *Postgrad Med J*; **946**:459–462.

Case 41

A 38-year-old man was brought to the emergency department by his wife. The patient was unable to give any history, was disorientated in place and time, and did not know why he was in hospital. His wife reported that he had become confused and drowsy during the day and had been complaining of headache. There was no past medical history and he worked as a labourer. He smoked 20 cigarettes a day and was not known to be taking any medication.

On examination, he was confused with a mini mental test score of 0/10 and was drowsy but easily roused. He was apyrexial and general examination appeared unremarkable except for the presence of multiple moles. There was no neck stiffness or photophobia, no papilloedema and no focal neurological deficit. The patient had a short-lived tonic clonic seizure in the emergency department.

Routine bloods and CXR were normal. The CT scan is shown in Fig. 41.1 (left and right images with and without contrast respectively).

Questions

41a) What does the CT scan show?

41b) Give a differential diagnosis for this CT scan appearance. What is the most likely diagnosis, based on the CT findings?

41c) How would you manage this patient?

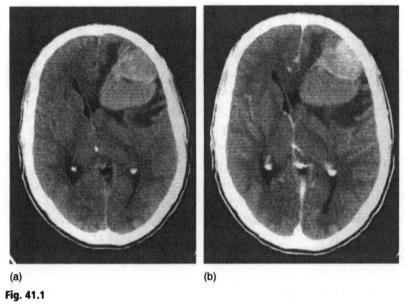

(a)   (b)

Fig. 41.1

Answers

41a) The CT scan shows a large left frontal space-occupying lesion with haemorrhage within it. There is extensive surrounding oedema.

41b) The differential diagnosis is of **primary or secondary brain tumour; metastatic melanoma** is the most likely.

Primary brain tumours including gliomas and meningiomas may haemorrhage. Secondary metastasis to the brain occurs most commonly in breast and lung cancer but is also seen in melanoma and other tumours. Haemorrhage is common in melanoma metastases but may occur with other metastatic tumours. There are no pathognomic features on CT/MRI that distinguish brain metastases from primary tumours but the differential diagnosis can be narrowed by new imaging techniques such as diffusion (see page 31) and perfusion weighted MRI and magnetic resonance spectroscopy although these are not generally used in routine clinical practice. The normal CXR together with the presence of multiple moles and an occupational history of manual work with probable significant sun exposure make the diagnosis of metastatic malignant melanoma the most likely.

41c) The management of the patient includes:

- Supportive therapy
- Steroids to reduce cerebral oedema
- Anticonvulsants for seizures
- Search for a primary tumour.

Further physical examination should be undertaken to look for a primary tumour source since this will help determine prognosis and possible radio-therapeutic or chemotherapeutic treatment. In this case, a suspicious 4.5 × 2.5cm irregularly outlined and pigmented skin lesion was found on the left chest. Subsequent dermatological review confirmed that this was a malignant melanoma and as likely primary.

Definitive therapy of **cerebral metastatic melanoma** depends on the clinical features of the individual patient, particularly the extent and location of metastasis. Patients with solitary brain metastases in the absence of systemic metastasis may obtain survival benefit from surgery and radiotherapy or stereotactic radiosurgery. Single brain metastases may also be removed to palliate symptoms. Whole brain radiotherapy may be used in patients with multiple or very large irresectable metas-tases for palliation of symptoms but appears not to improve survival and is associated with significant morbidity. Systemic therapy with new chemotherapeutic agents that cross the blood brain barrier is being considered. As yet there are no randomized trial data to determine the effectiveness of any of these therapies.

Further reading

Collins VP (2004). Brain tumours: classification and genes. J *Neurol Neurosurg Psychiatry*; 75 Suppl 2:ii2–11.

Douglas JG and Margolin K (2002). The treatment of brain metastases from malignant melanoma. *Semin Oncol*; 29(5):518–524.

Hildebrand J, De Witte O (1997). Treatment of tumours. *Curr Opin Neurol*; 10(6):459–463.

Rees J (2003). Advances in magnetic resonance imaging of brain tumours. *Curr Opin Neurol*; 16(6):643–650.

Tarhini AA, Agarwala SS (2004). Management of brain metastases in patients with melanoma. *Curr Opin Oncol*; 16(2):161–166.

Case 42

A 32-year-old man presented with severe drowsiness and confusion. He had been unwell for 2 weeks with headaches and a feeling as though he had 'worms in his head' followed by increasing sleepiness, causing him to be sent home from work. There were no other features on functional enquiry. There was no past medical history, recent travel abroad, or illegal drug taking. Alcohol intake was minimal. He was heterosexual and had had the same partner for the previous year. There was no family history of note.

On examination, he was of slim build, BM was 7.3mmol/L and general systems were normal. GCS was 13/15 and he was drowsy but rousable. He was disorientated in time, place and person. The rest of the neurological examination was normal within the limits of his compliance. Over the 2 weeks following admission, he remained extremely sleepy but rousable.

Investigation showed:

CXR and blood tests including U&E, LFT, TFT, CRP and ESR, FBC, glucose, Ca, PO_4 and serum ACE were normal. Thyroid autoantibodies were negative as were serological tests for Whipple's disease, Lyme disease and histoplasmosis.

MR brain imaging is shown in Fig. 42.1 (with thanks to Dr Camilla Buckley).

CSF examination showed 13 lymphocytes per ml and no polymorphs, glucose of 3.1g/dL (blood glucose 5.0g/dL), protein of 1.45g/dL and positive oligoclonal bands. There was no bacterial, viral or fungal growth, Indian ink stain and cryptococcal antigen were negative and cytological examination showed reactive T cells with a minority of B cells. No malignant cells were seen.

Questions

42a) How does sleep differ from coma?

42b) Give a differential diagnosis for excessive daytime sleepiness.

42c) Describe the MRI findings.

42d) What is the most likely cause of this patient's neurological syndrome? Give 4 other examples of this type of syndrome.

42e) Which other diagnoses would you have considered?

42f) What is the mechanism of this syndrome?

42g) How would you confirm your diagnosis?

42h) Given your diagnosis, what additional physical examination would you like to make in a young man of this age? What investigation would you request?

42i) What is the prognosis in patients with these types of syndromes?

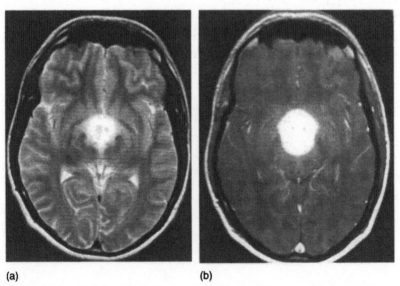

(a)   (b)

Fig. 42.1 T2-weighted axial MRI (a) showing high signal in the midline centred on the hypothalamus. There is striking enhancement on the corresponding axial contrast enhanced T1-weighted study (b).

Answers

42a) Patients who are asleep or sleepy can be roused sufficiently to respond to their environment whereas patients in coma cannot be roused in the same way. The EEG in normal sleep has several distinct and different EEG patterns. The EEG in coma is variable but in general does not resemble that of sleep.

42b) Neurological causes of daytime hypersomnolence (see list below) generally mediate their effects via interference with the ascending reticular activating arousal system and its projections to the posterior hypothalamus and thalamus. Lesions of this system usually cause coma rather than sleepiness. Occasionally tumours in the region of the III ventricle may be responsible. Narcolepsy has been reported with hypothalamus/ pituitary lesions, and cataplexy, hypnagogic hallucinations and sleep paralysis have been reported with rostral brainstem lesions. The non neurological and neurological causes of daytime sleepiness are listed below:

Non neurological

- *Metabolic encephalopathies:*
  - Hepatic, renal or respiratory failure
  - Electrolyte disturbances, hypoglycaemia
  - Hypothyroidism and acromegaly
  - Wernicke's encephalopathy (see page 18).
- *Toxins:*
  - Alcohol
  - Heavy metals (e.g. mercury see page 49).
- *Hypoxia*
- *Drugs*
- *Ventilatory disorders:*
  - Obstructive sleep apnoea
  - Central sleep apnoea
  - Central alveolar hypoventilation.
- *Psychiatric disorders*

Neurological

- *Structural lesions:*
  - Of the thalamus, hypothalamus, and brainstem.

- *CNS infections*:
  - Encephalitis lethargica (affects the posterior hypothalamic region)
  - Whipple's disease involving the hypothalamus (see page 48).
  - Sleeping sickness caused by *Trypanosoma gambiense* (characterized by fever and lymphadenopathy followed months or years later by excessive sleepiness, involuntary movements and sometimes coma and death).
- *Inflammatory conditions*:
  - Cerebral sarcoid (see page 273)
  - Langerhan's cell histiocytosis (see page 273)
  - MS.
- *Neurodegenerative conditions*:
  - Alzheimer's disease
  - Parkinson's disease
  - Multiple system atrophy
  - Myotonic dystrophy (both sleep apnoea and degeneration of the reticular activating system have been implicated).
- *Miscellaneous*:
  - Narcolepsy
  - Post trauma
  - Restless legs syndrome/periodic leg movement disorder
  - Paraneoplastic syndromes.

42c) The MRI brain shows T2-weighted hyperintensity in the hypothalamus and upper brainstem. These appearances are non-specific but possible causes include sarcoid, Langerhan's cell hystiocytosis, lymphoma, and paraneoplastic damage.

42d) The most likely diagnosis is of a **paraneoplastic syndrome**.

The brain imaging shows no evidence of a structural lesion and the laboratory investigations have ruled out most of the metabolic and endocrine causes of excessive sleepiness. There were no clinical features to suggest a neurodegenerative disorder, lymphoma, Langerhan's cell histiocytosis (see page 273) or sarcoid, although the latter diagnoses were not excluded by the investigation findings. Encephalitis lethargica was associated with extreme somnolence caused by extensive damage to the posterior hypothalamus, but this disorder is now rarely, if ever, seen.

The most likely diagnosis in this patient given the clinical features and the investigation results is a paraneoplastic syndrome causing a **brain-stem encephalitis**. Neurological paraneoplastic syndromes refer to a group of neurological disorders occurring in cancer patients, which are not associated with the direct effects of the cancer, cancer therapy, metabolic changes or vascular disease. Paraneoplastic disorders are associated with the presence of specific autoantibodies indicating a probable immunogenic cause but the antibodies themselves do not appear to be directly implicated in the neurological damage. Onset is usually subacute but may stabilize over weeks or months. The diagnosis is important because it implies the presence of what is usually an occult cancer and that may be curable. In addition, most paraneoplastic disorders result in severe disability but progression may sometimes be halted or reversed with treatment of the underlying tumour.

Examples of paraneoplastic syndromes include:

- Encephalopathy e.g. limbic encephalopathy (small cell lung cancer) (see Fig. 42.2), brain stem encephalopathy (testis-anti Ma2)

- Encephalomyelitis

- Cerebellar dysfunction (breast and ovary-anti-Yo, small cell lung-anti-Hu) eye movement disorders

- Retinopathy

- Neuropathy/radiculopathy/neuronopathy, including dorsal root ganglionitis (small cell lung cancer see page 262)

- Motor neuronopathy/motor neuron disease

- Neuromuscular dysfunction e.g. Lambert-Eaton myaesthenic syndrome (small cell lung cancer), myaesthenia gravis

- Myopathy/dermatomyositis (see page 22).

Some paraneoplastic syndromes (e.g. Lambert–Eaton) may be so characteristic as to allow a confident diagnosis on clinical grounds although such syndromes may occur in the absence of an associated cancer. Certain other syndromes are commonly associated with specific autoantibodies and particular types of cancer (see above) making the search for the underlying tumour easier. Although most patients have abnormalities restricted to one part of the nervous system, more diffuse patterns of involvement may be seen.

The CSF characteristically shows elevated protein, pleocytosis and oligoclonal bands as in the current patient although the protein and cell

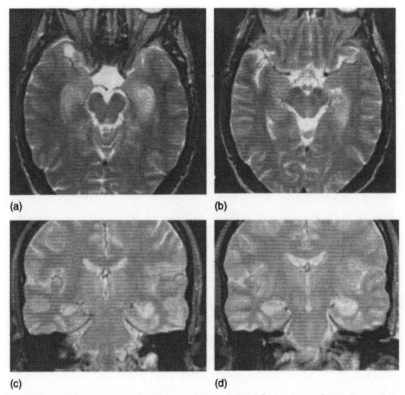

(a)

(b)

(c)

(d)

Fig. 42.2 Axial (upper images) and coronal T2-weighted (lower images) MRI in a patient with limbic encephalitis showing hyperintensity of the medial temporal lobes.

count may be normal. This patient showed anti-Ma2 antibody that is associated most commonly with testicular tumours but also with lung cancer and some other cancers e.g. breast and ovary. Anti-Ma2 is associated with limbic, hypothalamic, and brainstem encephalopathy with the majority of patients showing features of all three. Limbic encephalopathy causes short term memory deficits, confusion, cognitive decline, and psychomotor seizures. Hypothalamic damage causes excessive daytime sleepiness together with weight gain, hyperthermia, and endocrine abnormalities. Gelastic seizures and cataplexy may occur. Brainstem involvement is indicated by eye movement disorders, typically vertical gaze paresis, dysarthria, dysphagia, facial weakness, hearing loss, and facial numbness. Rarely, Parkinsonian syndromes and hypokinesis may be seen.

42e) The mechanism of paraneoplastic damage is unclear.

It is thought that onconeuronal antigens are shared between the tumour and particular nerve cells. The immune system directs a response against the tumour but also attacks the nerve cells sharing the specific tumour antigen leading to neurological abnormality. This immune response may be important in slowing tumour growth and would explain why many tumours associated with paraneoplastic syndromes are small and occult.

42f) Diagnosis depends on the identification where applicable, of a specific neurological syndrome together with the exclusion of alternative diagnoses and demonstration of paraneoplastic antibody together with the underlying tumour.

42g) The patient should be re-examined looking for an underlying tumour.

The majority of patients with a paraneoplastic syndrome develop neurological symptoms prior to tumour diagnosis. In a man of this age with a suspected paraneoplastic syndrome (and in the present case, detection of anti-Ma2 antibody), careful examination of the external genitalia together with testicular ultrasound should be performed.

42h) The prognosis depends on the underlying tumour and the extent of spread at presentation.

Young men with testicular cancer usually present when the disease is still very localized and complete cure is possible. In these cases, the prognosis is reasonable and improvement or even complete resolution of the neurological abnormalities may occur with tumour eradication. In older patients, in particular where the neoplastic disease cannot be cured, the prognosis is much worse and patients develop severe disability. There are reports of improvement with IVIg, plasma exchange, and immunosuppression but most patients are not helped by such treatments.

Further reading

Bataller L, Dalmau J (2003). Paraneoplastic neurologic syndromes. *Neurol Clin*; 21(1):221–247.

Dalmau J, Graus F, Villarejo A *et al* (2004). Clinical analysis of anti-Ma2-associated encephalitis. *Brain*; 127(8):1831–1844.

Dalmau JO, Posner JB (1999). Paraneoplastic syndromes. *Arch Neurol*; 56(4):405–488.

Case 43

A 67-year-old man presented with confusion and agitation. His wife explained that he had had 10 days of pain and swelling around the left eye and 2 weeks previously he had been refused elective correction of myopia on the grounds that the eye was infected. There was no past medical history, he lived with his wife, was a non-smoker, and did not drink alcohol.

On examination, there was marked left proptosis, and he was confused and drowsy with a GCS of 12/15. There was no focal neurology.

He was intubated and ventilated prior to CT scan of the brain and orbits. CT brain revealed sinusitis and a collection involving the left frontal, ethmoid, maxillary and sphenoid sinuses together with a breach in the posterior wall of the left frontal sinus and cerebritis of the left frontal lobe and left frontal oedema. He underwent surgery by the ENT surgeons to drain pus from the frontal and ethmoidal sinuses and the left eyelid. Two hours later, the right pupil became fixed and dilated, his intracranial pressure rose dramatically and the CT brain was repeated (see Fig. 43.1).

Questions

43a) What does the second CT brain (Fig. 43.1b) show?

43b) Why has he developed a fixed right pupil?

43c) What treatment is required?

43d) What are the possible complications of this condition?

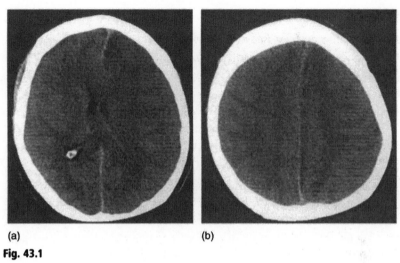

(a)   (b)

Fig. 43.1

Answers

43a) The CT scan shows **left subdural empyema.**

There is marked low density throughout both frontal lobes, more marked on the left, consistent with evolving cerebritis. There is an extensive subdural empyema (the hypodense area, see arrows on Fig. 43.2, the same image as shown in Fig. 43.1b) adjacent to the left parafalcine region causing local mass effect. The signs of subdural empyema on CT, seen as a hypodense rim around the surface of the brain, or adjacent to the falx as in the current case, may be very subtle and easily missed.

43b) The fixed right pupil indicates a right III nerve palsy. This is a false localizing sign caused by the III nerve being stretched by the cerebral oedema and local mass effect from the subdural empyema.

43c) He was given mannitol followed by urgent left frontal decompressive craniectomy, left frontal lobectomy, drainage of subdural empyema and insertion of ICP monitor. Polymicrobial flora of *Streptococcus milleri* and anaerobic species were grown from drained pus.

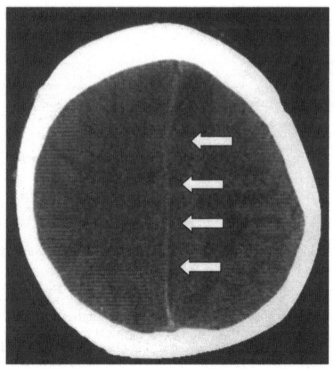

Fig. 43.2

In adults, subdural empyema most commonly results from extension of infection from the head usually the sinuses (in children, otitis media is the most common association, but it may also occur with meningitis). Infection of subdural haemorrhage and haematogenous spread from distant sources are also seen. Initial appearances on CT brain may be very subtle or even absent, and the diagnosis may be missed. Alternatively, a hypodense rim around the brain with mass effect, contrast enhancement and osteolyelitis may be present. MRI brain with gadolinium may be required in cases where the CT appearances are uncertain.

The clinical signs associated with subdural empyema are similar to those seen with cerebral abscess (see Fig. 43.3) and indicate a septic mass lesion. Headache (usually localized at onset) and fever occur early, followed by meningeal irritation, focal neurological signs and seizures. Causative organisms include β haemolytic streptococci, *Strep. milleri*, *Staphylococcus aureas*, *H. influenzae* and anaeorobes, and the subdural collection is often polymicrobial.

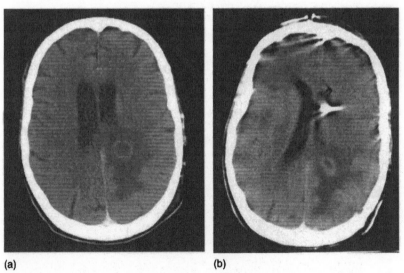

(a)   (b)

Fig. 43.3 CT brain with contrast showing a cerebral abscess in the deep white matter with ring enhancement and extensive surrounding oedema in a patient presenting with fever, headache, right hemiparesis and sensory disturbance, and generalized seizure on a background of sinusitis. The abscess is about to rupture into the lateral ventricle. Cerebral abscesses are more likely to occur in compromised tissue, for example; in infarcted tissue, at the junction of the grey and white matter, in patients with heart or lung disease, and in the immunocompromised patient

43d) The complications of subdural empyema include:

- Hydrocephalus
- Cerebral oedema
- CVT (see page 10)
- Cavernous sinus thrombosis
- Ventriculitis.

Further reading

Bernadini GL (2004). Diagnosis and management of brain abscess and subdural empyema. *Curr Neurol Neurosci Rep*; **4**(6):448–456. Review.

Dill SR, Cobbs CJ, McDonald CK (1995). Subdural empyema: analysis of 32 cases and review. *Clin Infect Dis*; **20**(2):372–386. Review.

Levy RM (1994). Brain abscess and subdural empyema. *Curr Opin Neurol*; **7**(3):223–228. Review.

Rich PM, Deasy NP, Jarosz JM (2000). Intracranial dural empyema. *Br J Radiol*; **73**(876):1329–1336. Review.

Case 44

A 44-year-old bartender presented with pain and numbness over the trunk and abdomen and numbness over the medial aspects of both arms, thighs and feet and ankles. Two weeks previously he had developed visible cervical lymphadenopathy, fever, malaise, rash, and headache. He was intermittently unsteady but he did not think his limbs were weak. He was homosexual and drank 1 bottle of spirits and smoked 60 cigarettes per day. He had recently moved from Africa to the UK. He was not taking any medication.

He was apyrexial with axillary and cervical lymphadenopathy and a maculopapular rash extending over the trunk with multiple excoriations. There was 2cm non-tender hepatomegaly. The neck was not stiff and he was alert and orientated. Cranial nerve examination revealed nystagmus on lateral gaze and rotatory nystagmus on upgaze. There was reduced hearing on the right. Upper limbs had normal tone and power but reduced reflexes on the right and reduced pin prick and temperature sensation in the C6–T2 distribution. There was radicular pain and hyperaesthesia in the T4–T6 distribution with accompanying reduced pin prick and temperature sensation bilaterally, but examination of the lower limbs was normal. Gait was slightly unsteady but Romberg's negative.

Investigations showed:

- CXR: normal
- CSF: opening pressure 18.5cm H_2O, 4 lymphocytes/mm^3, protein 0.54g/dL, glc 3.0mmol/L (blood 3.8mmol/L).

Questions

44a) Where are the lesions responsible for his neurological symptoms and signs?

44b) Give 3 conditions associated with the particular neurological lesion responsible for the sensory signs.

44c) What is the most likely diagnosis in this patient given all the clinical features, and why?

44d) How would you confirm your diagnosis?

44e) How would you treat this man?

Answers

44a) The clinical features of this case suggest that there are lesions of the:

- Brainstem (midbrain)
- Cerebellum/cerebellar connections
- Dorsal root ganglia.

Diplopia and nystagmus are caused by an abnormality of the midbrain or the cranial nerves controlling eye movements and balance (III, IV, VI, and VIII). The presence of rotatory nystagmus on upgaze suggests a central cause. Reduced hearing is caused by abnormalities of the VIII nerve or its central connections. The upper limb signs are sensory without a motor component and are mainly dermatomal. Together with the reduced upper limb reflexes on the right and the dermatomal pain in the trunk, this indicates pathology of the sensory part of the nerve roots in multiple sites and would be consistent with a dorsal root ganglionopathy. A radiculopathy might be expected to produce motor as well as sensory signs and a sensory peripheral neuropathy would not have a dermatomal pattern. Unsteadiness of gait together with the nystagmus and negative Romberg test suggests a disorder of the cerebellum or its connections.

44b) In contrast to axonal or demyelinating sensory neuropathies, sensory neuronopathy where the dorsal root ganglion is the site of pathology is a rare syndrome. Causes include:

- Paraneoplastic syndrome (see page 252) e.g. associated with small cell cancer of the lung (at least two-thirds of cases) in which all sensory modalities are usually involved and pseudoathetoid movements may occur
- Sjorgren's syndrome
- Heavy metal poisoning
- Drugs e.g. cisplatin
- Infectious/parainfectious: CMV, HIV, Miller–Fisher syndrome
- Friedrich's ataxia.

Differentiation from sensory neuropathy clinically may be impossible, especially as there may be co-existent peripheral neuropathy. Nerve conduction studies show global reduction or loss of sensory nerve action potentials.

Sensory ganglioneuronopathy is a characteristic paraneoplastic syndrome seen in association particularly with small cell lung cancer and may precede the diagnosis of cancer by months, or even years.

Patients present with pain, paraesthesia, ataxic gait, pseudoathetoid movements, and reduced or absent reflexes. Changes may be asymmetrical and both proximal and distal body sites may be involved. It is associated with anti-Hu antibody. There is variable involvement of motor nerves and central regions. However, this patient's acute inflammatory illness immediately prior to the onset of neurological symptoms makes this diagnosis unlikely.

Sensory ganglionopathy is the distinctive neuropathy of Sjorgren's syndrome accounting for 10–20% of neuropathies seen in this condition and may antedate diagnosis by some months, or even years. Other inflammatory conditions such as connective tissue disease, vasculitides and sarcoid may cause fever, lymphadenopathy and rash together with central or peripheral nervous system disease but sensory ganglionopathies have not been reported to our knowledge.

Systemic symptoms may occur with drugs that may cause a sensory neuronopathy but this patient was not taking any medication prior to presentation.

44c) The most likely diagnosis is **primary HIV infection (HIV seroconversion)**.

The clinical features of this case suggest an inflammatory process with associated nervous system involvement and in a homosexual man from Africa, HIV seroconversion must be considered. HIV seroconversion (formation of antibody) lasts days to weeks and occurs 2–6 weeks after exposure to the HIV virus. Symptoms accompany seroconversion in 40–90% of infected subjects and are EBV-like comprising fever, pharyngitis, weight loss, night sweats, lymphadenopathy, myalgia, headache, nausea and diarrhoea, rash, and mucosal ulcers. There may be accompanying leukopaenia, thrombocytopaenia and mild transaminitis. The differential diagnosis of acute HIV infection includes:

- Viral infection:
  - CMV
  - EBV
  - Rubella
  - Hepatitis
  - Influenza
  - Herpes simplex.
- Bacterial infection:
  - Lyme disease
  - Syphilis

- Rickettsia
- Gonococcus
- Streptococcus.
- Non infectious:
  - Connective tissue
  - Drugs
  - Vasculitides
  - Adult Still's disease.

Diagnosis of HIV seroconversion is often difficult owing to the non-specific nature of the symptoms but early recognition may prevent unknowing transmission of HIV during the accompanying phase of high-level viraemia and may enable early potentially disease-modifying treatment. Diagnostic pointers towards HIV seroconversion include rash, mucosal ulcers, generalized lymphadenopathy and neurologic abnormalities. **EBV** rarely causes a rash (unless amoxycillin is given) or diarrhoea but is associated with jaundice in 10% (see page 78) (jaundice is not seen in primary HIV infection), tonsillar exudates, and cervical lymphadenopthy. In the patient described above, the presence of a ganglioneuronopathy narrowed the differential diagnosis since most of the disorders that may mimic HIV seroconversion (see above) are not reported to cause a ganglioneuronopathy. EBV (and HIV) may be associated with **Guillain–Barré syndrome** (see page 76).

Neurological abnormalities associated with HIV seroconversion are many and include:

- Aseptic meningitis
- Demyelinating syndromes resembling MS
- VII nerve palsy
- Guillain–Barré-like syndrome
- Radiculopathy, ganglioneuronopathy
- Myositis.

Neurologic syndromes may also occur at later points in the course of HIV infection (see page 87) through HIV itself (meningitis, encephalopathy) or secondary pathologies (TB, opportunistic infection, lymphoma). A distal symmetrical predominantly sensory painful polyneuropathy is the most common peripheral neuropathy in patients with low CD4 counts but CIDP and mononeuritis multiplex may also occur. CMV infection, herpes zoster, syphilis and lymphomatous root infiltration may cause radiculopathy.

44d) HIV antibodies are often not present at the time of presentation. HIV viral load should be measured together with follow-up antibody testing.

44e) Initiation of therapy in patients with primary HIV infection is controversial.

The British HIV Association guidelines recommend treatment only for relief of symptoms. In the US, consideration of treatment is recommended in those who receive a diagnosis ≤ 6 months after infection. Studies have shown immunologic benefits from antiretroviral therapy up to 3–4 months after infection but long-term effects are unknown.

Further reading

Berger JR, Levy RM (eds) (1997). *AIDS and the nervous system (2nd edition)*. Philadelphia: Lippincott-Raven.

Brew BJ (2003). The peripheral nerve complications of human immunodeficiency virus (HIV) infection. *Muscle Nerve*; 28:542–552.

Elder G, Dalakas M, Pezeshkpour G, Sever J (1986). Ataxic neuropathy due to ganglioneuritis after probable acute human immunodeficiency virus infection. *Lancet*; ii:1275–1276.

Kassutto S and Rosenberg ES (2004). Primary HIV type 1 infection. *Clin Infect Dis*; 38(10):1447–1453.

Kuntzer T, Antoine JC, Steck AJ (2004). Clinical features and pathophysiological basis of sensory neuronopathies (ganglionopathies). *Muscle Nerve*; 30(3):255–268.

Price RW (1996). Neurological complications of HIV infection. *Lancet*; 348:445–452.

Case 45

A 79-year-old woman described a 1-month history of gradually progressive unpleasant tingling in the hands together with problems fastening buttons and gripping small objects, difficulty walking and unsteadiness. This was associated with short-term memory loss over the preceding few months: she reported difficulty remembering names and playing bridge, although longer-term memory was intact. General examination was unremarkable. MMSE was 25/30 with deficits in short-term recall and orientation. There was small muscle wasting in the hands with mild weakness. Tone was increased in the legs with clonus at the ankles and mild bilateral pyramidal weakness. Reflexes were brisk except for the ankle jerks, which were absent. The left plantar reflex was upgoing. Vibration and position sense were absent at the ankles with definite Rombergism. In addition, there was finger nose ataxia, dysdiadochokinesis and ataxic gait.

Investigations showed:

- HB 12.5g/dL, MCV 100fL, WCC 6.0×10^9/L, Plt 259×10^9/L, Na 138mmol/L, K 3.6mmol/L, urea 6mmol/L, Cr 124μmol/L.

Questions

45a) What is the most likely diagnosis and why?

45b) What else would you like to examine clinically?

45c) What is the most common cause of this condition? Give 3 other causes.

45d) How would you confirm your diagnosis?

45e) What is the prognosis?

Answers

45a) The most likely diagnosis is **vitamin B12 deficiency**.

The clinical features of this case imply abnormalities in several different areas of the nervous system:

- Cognitive impairment indicating disease of the cerebral hemispheres

- Increased tone in the legs with an upgoing left plantar indicating cord pathology or bilateral pathology in the descending motor pathways in the brain

- Wasting of the small hand muscles indicating a peripheral neuropathy, anterior horn cell pathology or cord abnormality at the cervical/T1 level

- Absent ankle jerks indicating peripheral neuropathy

- Tingling in the hands indicating sensory neuropathy, radiculopathy, neuronopathy, or disease of the central sensory pathways

- Impairment of vibration/position sense in the legs indicating a sensory polyneuropathy, neuronopathy or disease of the dorsal columns

- Gait and upper limb ataxia that could not be explained on the basis of a sensory ataxia indicating disease of the cerebellum or its connections.

The blood tests show a macrocytosis. Taken together the most likely diagnosis is B12 deficiency. B12 deficiency causes damage to the brain, spinal cord (dorsal and lateral columns) and peripheral nerves. It presents with paraesthesia in the hands and feet in the majority of patients and weakness and unsteadiness of gait are the next most frequent symptoms. Mental slowness, confusion, depression, and hallucinations may occur and may be the presenting features.

On examination, there are usually signs of both peripheral nerve and cord involvement with or without cognitive changes. Loss of vibration and position sense in the legs is a consistent finding caused by dorsal column damage. Reflex abnormalities are variable: reflexes may be reduced or absent in the legs if there is associated peripheral neuropathy but may otherwise be brisk. The legs are spastic secondary to damage to the descending motor pathways in the lateral spinal cord. Cerebellar and brainstem abnormalities may be present. Optic atrophy, visual loss and scotomata are occasionally seen. In this patient, there was wasting of the small muscles of the hand which is not usually seen in B12 deficiency but in a patient of this age there may be coexistent cervical myelopathy.

Nerve conduction studies show small or absent sural nerve sensory potentials in 80% indicating an axonal polyneuropathy but features of demyelination may also be present. Visual and somatosensory evoked potentials are frequently abnormal. Pathological specimens show damage to the brain, spinal cord and peripheral nerves with demyelination and axonal loss in the dorsal columns of the thoracic cord extending to the lateral cord and the rest of the spinal white matter in severe cases. Demyelination also occurs in the cerebral white matter and the optic nerves. The peripheral nerves show evidence of both axonal loss and demyelination.

45b) Opthalmological examination including fundoscopy for optic atrophy and visual field measurement should be performed looking for the visual abnormalities described above.

45c) The most common cause of B12 deficiency is pernicious anaemia (defective intrinsic factor production by gastric parietal cells). Other causes include:

- Surgical resection of the terminal ileum
- Veganism
- Bacterial overgrowth
- Fish tapeworm infestation (dithylbothium latum)
- Coeliac disease, tropical sprue, Whipple's disease
- Chronic gastritis, gastrectomy.

45d) FBC and film should be performed to look for macrocytosis and hyper-segmented neutrophils.

Anaemia may not be present at the time of neurological presentation. Serum B12 should be measured together with antibodies to gastric parietal cells and intrinsic factor (elevated in 60–90%). B12 levels may be normal in deficiency states particularly in hepatic or myeloproliferative disorders and conversely may be low in pregnancy in the absence of deficiency. A therapeutic trial of B12 may be useful where there is uncertainty.

45e) Replacement therapy should be instituted without delay. A variable degree of recovery occurs mainly over the first six months but improvement may continue up to one year. In general recently acquired symptoms respond better than long established abnormalities, hence the importance of early diagnosis and treatment.

Further reading

Skeen MB (2002). Neurological manifestations of gastrointestinal disease. *Neurol Clin*; 20(1):195–225,vii.

Case 46

A 32-year-old man described a 9-month history of retro-orbital pain, left fixed pupil, drooping of the left eyelid, and double vision with intermittent left temporal headache which was worse at night. He also described a dry mouth and drinking between 4 and 10L per day. Examination revealed a left pupil that was 2mm larger than the right and there was a squint with the left eye looking downwards and laterally together with a left ptosis. There was double vision in all directions of gaze except looking down and to his left. The rest of the neurological examination was normal.

Investigations showed:

- Plasma osmolality 304mosmol/kg (278–305mosmol/kg)
- Urine osmolality 63mosmol/kg (380–1000mosmol/kg)
- WCC 21.7×10^9 L (neutrophils 88%)
- ESR 34mm/h, CRP < 8g/dL.

Questions

46a) Where is the neurological lesion? What is the commonest cause of this where there is associated pain?

46b) Suggest 3 possible causes for a similar painless lesion, and explain the reason for the pupillary sparing that is often seen in such cases.

46c) What is the explanation for the other clinical features and the investigation results?

46d) The MRI scan showed infiltrative pathology affecting the hypothalamus. Give 3 possible diagnoses that would explain the clinical features of this case.

46e) What further investigations would you perform?

Answers

46a) The clinical findings indicate a **lesion of the left III cranial nerve**.

The left pupillary enlargement, left ptosis, and squint with the left eye deviated downwards and laterally together with double vision in all directions of gaze except when looking down and to the left suggest a left III nerve lesion. In this patient, there was associated retro-orbital pain. Painful extraocular palsies are nearly always surgical rather than medical in aetiology and require urgent investigation. The commonest cause of a painful III nerve palsy is an aneurysm of the posterior communicating artery (see Fig. 46.1) which runs parallel to the III nerve after the latter's exit from between the cerebral peduncles. The presence of such an aneurysm should prompt urgent neurosurgical referral.

46b) Painless III nerve palsies usually have a medical cause, examples include diabetes mellitus, syphilis, and sarcoid.

In such 'medical' causes of a III nerve palsy, the pupil is often not involved as the parasympathetic nerve bundle subserving pupillary constriction runs superficially within the III nerve and has a separate vascular supply. The III nerve nucleus may be affected by pathology in the midbrain but in this case there are usually other accompanying brainstem signs.

46c) The osmolality and fluid balance abnormalities suggest diabetes insipidus.

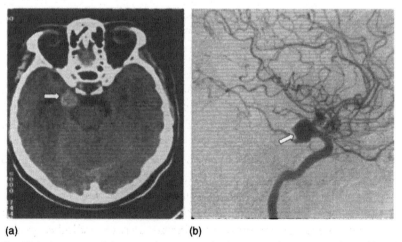

(a)   (b)

Fig. 46.1 Aneurysm of the posterior communicating artery shown on CT brain (a) and catheter angiography (b) (with thanks to Dr James Byrne).

The large oral fluid intake together with the low urine osmolality and high normal plasma osmolality in a patient with intracranial pathology suggest diabetes insipidus. Diabetes insipidus is caused by lack of ADH secretion or peripheral insensitivity to this hormone (nephrogenic diabetes insipidus). Intracranial causes include Sheehan's syndrome (pituitary infarction associated with pregnancy), hypothalamic-pituitary surgery, trauma, ischaemia, space occupying lesions including metastases (especially breast), infiltrative conditions such as sarcoid, and intracranial infections including TB and meningococcus.

46d) The differential diagnosis of an infiltrative disorder affecting the hypothalamus and pituitary gland together with a III nerve palsy and diabetes insipidus includes:

- Sarcoid
- Langerhan's cell histiocytosis (histiocytosis X)
- TB.

Sarcoid is a multisystem granulomatous disorder of unknown aetiology. Typical presentation is with hilar lymphadenopathy, lung infiltrates, skin and eye lesions. Neurological involvement occurs in 5% and is the presenting feature in 50% of these patients. Inflammation occurs primarily in the leptomeninges and spreads to involve the brain, cord and peripheral nerves. The neurological manifestations are diverse and include cranial neuropathies, (VII being the most frequently affected often bilaterally, see page 92), hypothalamic-pituitary disorders, peripheral neuropathy, and myopathy. The diagnosis is usually based on characteristic clinical features in a patient with systemic sarcoid on clinical, imaging or histopathological findings but may be difficult in patients with isolated CNS disease.

Langerhan's cell histiocytosis (histiocytosis X) is a poorly-understood disorder in which dysfunctional populations of Langerhan's cells (derived from haemopoietic cells in the bone marrow) are present in areas of tissue involvement. Children are most commonly affected but it may occur at any age. Single or multisystem organ involvement may be seen including osteolytic bone lesions, skin rash, anaemia and pancytopaenia, hepatomegaly, lung cysts, and malabsorption. In the CNS, the hypothalamic pituitary axis is most commonly affected and diabetes insipidus is the most common presentation. Diagnosis requires tissue biopsy. Treatment options include steroids, radiotherapy and chemotherapy although there are no systematic trials and spontaneous resolution may occur.

Diabetes insipidus may occur with intracranial infection, particularly TB, which may also cause an infiltrative appearance on MRI. However, the clinical features of this case do not otherwise suggest TB.

46e) CXR, serum ACE, brain biopsy (if no other abnormal tissue seen).

Further reading

Burnol DJ, Watson JD, Roddie M, *et al* (1992). Langerhans' cell histiocytosis and the nervous system. *J Neurol*; **239**(6):345–350.

Grois NG, Favara BE, Mostbeck,GH *et al* (1994). Central nervous system disease in Langerhans cell histiocytosis. *Br J Cancer Suppl*; **23**:S24–28.

Hasegawa K, Mitomi T, Kowa H, *et al* (1993). A clinico-pathological study of adult histiocytosis X involving the brain. *J Neurol Neurosurg Psychiatry*; **56**(9):1008–1012.

Murialdo G, Tamagno G (2002). Endocrine aspects of neurosarcoidosis. *J Endocrinol Invest*; **25**:650–662.

Zajicek JP (2000). Neurosarcoidosis. *Curr Opci Neurol*; **13**(3):323–325.

Case 47

Case A An 81-year-old man presented with an 18-month history of progressive difficulty walking and painful paraesthesiae in the soles of his feet. His referral was prompted by the development of urinary urgency with mild incontinence and perineal numbness for the preceding 2 months. He described acute excacerbations of his symptoms when his legs became weaker and 'like jelly', often occurring after gardening or a hot bath. There was no weight loss and he felt otherwise well. He had a 30-year history of low/mid thoracic back pain that had begun mildly but had progressed very gradually over the years such that it was severe enough at times to interrupt his sleep at the time of presentation. Plain X-rays of the back performed some years previously, had shown nil of note. There was no other past medical history. He was on no medication other than analgesia for the back pain. He was a non-smoker and took little alcohol.

On examination, general systems were unremarkable, as were the cranial nerves and the upper limbs. In the lower limbs there was no wasting and the tone was increased, there was bilateral weakness, pathologically brisk reflexes, bilateral upgoing plantars, and he was only able to walk a few steps with a frame owing to marked spasticity. There was a sensory level at T6.

Case B A 60-year-old medical secretary presented with a 3-week history of lower limb symptoms beginning with bilateral calf discomfort and numb feet. One week later, she noticed leg weakness, difficulty climbing stairs, and mild lower back pain. There were no bladder or bowel symptoms. There was a past history of breast cancer diagnosed the previous year for which she had received surgery, chemotherapy and radiotherapy.

On examination, the cranial nerves and upper limbs were normal. There was bilateral foot drop and she was unable to stand on her toes. There was reduced tone in both lower limbs and mild weakness bilaterally. Sensation was reduced to pin prick over L4, L5, and partial S1. Joint position and vibration were preserved. There was no sacral sensory loss. Reflexes were normal in the upper limbs, absent at the knees and preserved at the ankles and plantars were mute.

Nerve conduction studies and EMG were normal apart from showing reduced voluntary activation. The CXR and MRI are shown in Figs. 47.1 and 47.2 respectively.

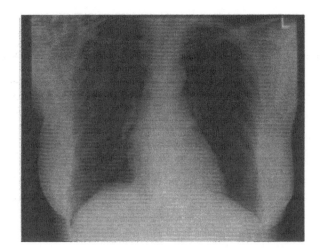

Fig. 47.1

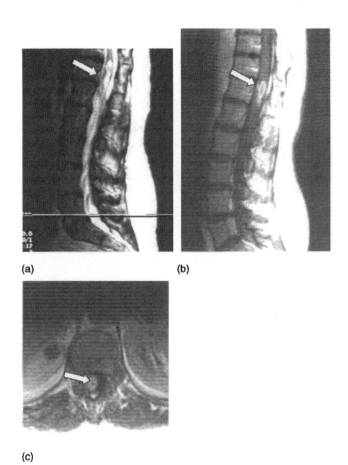

(a)

(b)

(c)

Fig. 47.2

Questions

47a) Where is the lesion in each case (the lesion is indicated by the arrows on the MRI from case B)?

47b) What is the most likely diagnosis in case A?

47c) How would you confirm the diagnosis? What is the treatment?

47d) What does the CXR from case B show? What is the most likely diagnosis?

Answers

47a) The features of both cases suggest spinal cord pathology:

- Above T6 in case A
- At the conus in case B.

In case A, the clinical features suggest a cord lesion above T6. In case B, there are sensory and motor symptoms and signs in the legs with reduced tone and absent knee jerks with preserved ankle jerks. The normal nerve conduction studies show no evidence of a peripheral neuropathy (in which one would expect loss of ankle as well as knee jerks) but the lack of upper motor neuron signs indicates that the pathology must involve the lumbosacral nerve roots (L2–S2). The symmetrical presentation makes a plexopathy unlikely. The T2-weighted sagittal MRI shows a high signal lesion in the conus (the most inferior part of the spinal cord). The contrast enhanced T1 (sagittal and axial) shows irregular enhancement within the cord consistent with a metastatic deposit.

In general, the clinical features of spinal cord lesions depend on whether the lesions are located outside or inside the cord and the spinal level at which they are situated, but it should be noted that the clinical presentation may be atypical. Cord compression from extrinsic (outside the cord substance) lesions tends to cause primarily motor symptoms at first, the reasons for which are unclear, although there may be sensory change at the level of the lesion, particularly if the lesion arises from a nerve root. In early cases, the patient initially complains of heaviness of the legs and dragging of the feet and there is a mild spastic paraparesis on examination, although hyperacute progression to complete paralysis may occur in e.g. vascular damage. Impending irreversible cord damage is indicated by the onset of micturition disturbance or sensory symptoms. Typically, sensory symptoms start with tingling in the feet that ascends to 2 or 3 segments below the actual level of compression.

Intrinsic (intramedullary–within the cord) cord lesions in contrast tend to cause sensory symptoms initially owing to the course of the pain and temperature pathways within the central spinal cord. A lesion e.g. glioma or syrinx in the central cord will irritate pain and temperature fibres as they cross the cord, initially only at the level of the lesion. In the cervical cord, a unilateral or bilateral Horner's syndrome may occur. It is only when the cord becomes markedly expanded that long tract signs occur with brisk reflexes and extensor plantars. Gradual involvement of the spinothalamic tract causes descending spinothalamic sensory loss (fibres from successively more proximal parts of the body enter centrally and push the existing fibres outwards such that the upper limb fibres lie centrally in the tract at the cervical level with the lower limb fibres lying more laterally). In the final stages of this process, only the fibres from the sacral area survive (since these travel most peripherally in the spinothalamic tract) and there is sacral sparing, a rare but diagnostic feature of an intrinsic cord lesion.

It should be noted that the spinal cord terminates at the level of the L1/L2 vertebrae leaving the nerve roots from T12–S5 to descend within the spinal canal as the cauda equina. Lesions in the spinal canal at any level below T10 can cause a cauda equina syndrome. In the adult, there are 3 main clinical pictures. The lateral cauda equina syndrome is usually caused by a neurofibroma. For example, such a lesion on the L4 nerve root would cause anterior thigh pain, quadriceps wasting, weakness of inversion of the foot and an absent knee jerk. If the lesion is high and lateral to the cord, there may be pyramidal signs below the lesion ie brisk ankle jerks and an extensor plantar and spincter disturbance from cord compression. Midline cauda equina lesions may occur from within the cord or from outside. Those from within (conus lesion) tend to cause S5 root damage initially and progress causing sacral pain, micturition difficulty, and impotence. Later there is loss of ankle jerks and weakness of the L5 and S1 muscle groups. Midline cauda equina lesions from without generally cause bilateral lumbar and sacral root lesions. Root pain in the L2, L3, S2, or S3 distribution should be regarded with suspicion as a sinister cause is likely whereas pain in the L4, L5 or S1 distribution is more likely to be caused by disc disease. It should be noted however, that the correlation between actual lesion location and the clinical findings in cauda equina/conus pathology is not exact.

Spinal cord lesions may be intramedullary (within the cord substance) or extramedullary (outside the cord). The latter are intra- or extradural. Examples of extradural lesions include chordomas, sarcomas and intervertebral discs. Intradural lesions include meningiomas and neurofibromas. Metastatic spinal tumours (20–30% of spinal tumours in adults) are usually extradural rather than intramedullary. Intramedullary lesions include gliomas, ependymomas, syrinx, and metastatic deposits. Vascular lesions such as arteriovenous malformations, may occur within the cord, dura or vertebral bodies and cause symptoms through compression, vascular steal, or haemorrhage.

All patients with symptoms suggestive of cord pathology should have full physical examination, including of the breasts and prostate, and a CXR. In the absence of a sensory level, the cervical spine and thoracic spine including at least the L1 vertebra should be imaged in spastic paraparesis. In patients with a sensory level in whom initial imaging is negative, imaging of all spinal levels above the previously imaged level should be undertaken since the sensory level may lie several levels below the actual cord lesion. In patients with low back pain, lumbar root pain and mixed upper and lower signs in the legs, the region from T10 to L3 is the most important to image. If rectal or genital pain is present then the sacrum should be included but the spinal column to T10 must be imaged as well.

47b) The diagnosis in case A was **dural arteriovenous malformation (AVM)**.

In case A, there is a very long history of back pain. The location of the pain in the mid-to-low thoracic region coinciding with the likely level of cord pathology, together with its gradual increase in severity, suggests that it is related to the causative lesion. The fact that the lesion appears to have been present for 30 years suggests a benign cause. An intrinsic cord lesion is very unlikely to be the cause of this patient's symptoms because of the late development of neurological symptoms and a benign extrinsic cord lesion or bony lesion would be more likely. The presence of excacerbations in this patient's symptoms related to exercise and hot baths suggests a vascular cause and this together with the long history of back pain is consistent with spinal dural AVM (see below).

47c) The diagnosis of spinal dural AVM is made on MR imaging of the cord with gadolinium followed by spinal angiography. Treatment is with embolization or surgery.

In case A, MRI showed enlarged intradural vessels and increased signal in the cord. A dural AVM arising from the T9 radicular artery was confirmed on angiogram and treated by embolisation, with initial improvement in his symptoms. After 1 month, the symptoms recurred and he underwent surgery in which multiple feeder vessels were ligated.

Spinal AVMs are most common in middle-aged and elderly men and present with back pain (42%) and leg weakness. Acute onset syndromes or sudden acute deterioration may occur. Acute exacerbations may be related to exercise, posture, hot baths, pregnancy, Valsalva manoeuvres, and lumbar puncture or angiography. Increased venous pressure has been proposed as the mechanism by which neurologic dysfunction occurs: spinal cord biopsies show hypocellular white matter, vascular sclerosis and gliosis of white matter. MRI has 85–90% sensitivity and 82–100% specificity and shows increased cord signal on T2-weighted images together with flow voids in the intradural space, and enhancement of the cord margin and in the intradural space (serpentine pattern) with gadolinium.

47c) The CXR shows a **right lung lesion.** The most likely diagnosis in case B is a **cauda equina/conus lesion from metastatic breast cancer.**

In case B, the CXR shows a lesion in the right lung consistent with a metastasis likely to be from the breast cancer diagnosed the previous year. Thus, the most likely neurological diagnosis is a conus lesion from metastatic breast cancer. She was given palliative treatment including dexamethosone and radiotherapy.

Further reading

Aminoff MJ, Logue V (1974). Clinical features of spinal vascular malformations. *Brain*; **97**(1):197–210.

Schiff D, O'Neill BP (1996). Intramedullary spinal cord metastases: clinical features and treatment outcome. *Neurology*; **47**(4):906–912.

Schiff D, O'Neill BP, Suman VJ (1997). Spinal epidural metastasis as the initial manifestation of malignancy: clinical features and diagnostic approach. *Neurology*; **49**:452–456.

Song JK, Vinuela F, Gobin YP *et al* (2001). Surgical and endovascular treatment of spinal dural arteriovenous fistulas: long-term disability assessment and prognostic factors. *J Neurosurg Spine*; **94**(2):199–204.

Case 48

A 33-year-old woman presented with a 1-week history of severe pain in the right ear radiating to the jaw. Three days after the onset of the pain she had developed right facial weakness with associated tinnitus, hearing loss, and vertigo, with a tendency to fall to the left. On examination, there was a right lower motor neuron VII palsy with sensorineural hearing loss on the right. The gait was unsteady and she veered to the left when trying to walk.

Questions

48a) What is the most likely diagnosis and its cause?

48b) Describe the neural pathways involved in this condition with reference to the associated clinical features.

48c) What is the most common cause of an isolated lower motor neuron VII palsy? Which conditions are associated with bilateral lower motor neuron VII palsies?

48d) What treatment is available, if any, for this patient's condition?

Answers

48a) The most likely diagnosis is **Ramsay Hunt syndrome** or herpes zoster auricularis.

Ramsay Hunt syndrome is caused by herpes zoster damage to the VII cranial nerve. The syndrome was first described by Ramsay Hunt in 1907, who noted facial palsy associated with a vesicular eruption on the hard palate, anterior two thirds of the tongue and/or the external auditory meatus. Vesicles do not always occur (zoster sine herpete) or they may occur late but the presence of severe pain around the ear is highly suggestive of herpes zoster infection. Facial paralysis is maximal after about a week. VZV DNA has been demonstrated in aural secretions and in vesicular fluid and is associated with a rise in VZV antibody. It is the second most common cause of non-traumatic facial palsy after Bell's palsy.

Ramsay Hunt's observations led to a clearer understanding of the sensory functions of the VII nerve. The facial nerve supplies motor fibres to the face but also receives sensory fibres from the pinna and external auditory meatus (cutaneous), and the anterior two thirds of the tongue and the hard palate (taste) and supplies parasympathetic fibres to the salivary and lacrimal glands. The cell bodies of the sensory fibres of the VII nerve lie within the geniculate ganglion within the facial canal of the petrous temporal bone. Vesicular eruption on the hard palate, anterior tongue or external auditory meatus is caused by herpes zoster virus reactivation in the geniculate ganglion. Ramsay Hunt noted that VIII nerve features (tinnitus, hearing loss, nausea, vomiting, vertigo, and nystagmus) often accompanied the facial palsy, and are explained by the close proximity of the VIII nerve to the geniculate ganglion. Occasionally, there is an associated glossopharyngeal or vagal neuropathy presumably from viral spread within the mouth where the VII, IX and X cranial nerves are all represented consistent with their development from the same brachial arch.

48c) **Bell's palsy** is the most common cause of an isolated lower motor neuron VII palsy.

Bell's palsy may be associated with discomfort or mild pain around the ear, often preceding the facial palsy, but severe pain is uncommon and the VIII nerve is typically not affected. Severe pain or VIII nerve involvement thus suggests Ramsay Hunt syndrome. Paralysis is usually maximal 2 days after onset. The major cause of Bell's palsy is reactivation of latent herpes simplex type I: the presence of viral DNA within the facial nerve during facial paralysis has been demonstrated using PCR. It accounts for three quarters of non-traumatic facial palsy and there is a higher incidence in pregnancy.

Recurrent or bilateral facial nerve palsy should prompt investigation for **diabetes, sarcoid** (see page 273) and **Lyme disease** (see page 92); the latter should always be excluded in endemic areas. Bilateral facial nerve palsy also occurs in **Guillain–Barré syndrome** (see page 76) and **HIV** infection (see page 263). Slowly progressive paralysis with other associated cranial neuropathies suggests the possibility of a neoplastic process. As a general rule, lesions proximal to, or at, the geniculate ganglion tend to affect taste and lacrimation, whereas lesions distal to the geniculate ganglion produce, muscle weakness only.

48d) Facial palsy secondary to herpes zoster infection has a worse prognosis than Bell's palsy.

In untreated patients, only 10% of patients with complete paralysis and around two-thirds with partial paralysis recover completely. In Bell's palsy, approximately 70% of complete palsies and 95–100% of partial palsies recover in 6 weeks. Prognosis is worse in pregnancy, age over 60-years, or if there is associated hypertension or diabetes.

Eye care, including eye drops and nocturnal eye ointment together with artificial closure of the eye if necessary, should be given to prevent corneal complications. Treatment with steroids and antiviral agents has been shown to improve outcome in patients with Ramsay Hunt syndrome and Bell's palsy, and to prevent progression to complete paralysis. Early treatment (within 72 hours) is considerably more effective than late treatment (after 7 days).

Further reading

Holland NJ and Weiner GM (2004). Recent developments in Bell's palsy. *BMJ*; **329**:553–557.
Sweeney CJ and Gilden DH (2001). Ramsay Hunt syndrome. *JNNP*; **71**:149–154.

Case 49

A 47-year-old female driving instructor presented with left leg pain and numbness. A couple of weeks previously she had received amoxycillin for sinusitis and this was followed 4 days later by an itchy rash over the forehead and scalp which extended over the back. She was given a course of steroids to which the rash responded but reappeared after cessation of the steroids. Subsequently, she experienced sharp pains like hot needles in the left foot, and the index and ring finger of the left hand became numb. Past medical history revealed several previous episodes of sinusitis and late onset asthma that had been difficult to control, requiring multiple steroid courses. She had lost 21lb (9.5kg) over the previous year but there were no other symptoms of note.

General systems examination revealed a wheeze but nil else. Upper limb examination showed weakness of abductor pollicis brevis, flexor digitorum profundus and wrist flexion on the left and reduced sensation over the lateral 3.5 digits. Lower limb examination showed decreased power of left ankle dorsiflexion and eversion and there was a left foot drop. Sensation was reduced over the left anterior leg and dorsum of the foot. Limb reflexes were intact.

Questions

49a) What are the neurological lesions causing this woman's symptoms? What is this called? Give 4 conditions associated with this neurological syndrome.

49b) What is the most likely diagnosis in this woman? Describe the characteristic clinical features of this condition.

49c) What 4 further tests would you like to perform to confirm your diagnosis?

49d) What are the other neurological manifestations of this condition?

49e) How would you treat this condition?

Answers

49a) There are left median and left common peroneal nerve lesions.

The neurological findings indicate lesions of the left median nerve causing weakness of thumb abduction, finger and wrist flexion and sensory change over the lateral three and a half digits and of the left common peroneal nerve causing foot drop and sensory change over the anterior thigh leg and foot. This involvement of multiple peripheral nerves is termed mononeuritis multiplex.

Causes of mononeuritis multiplex include:

- Axonal:
  - Vasculitis
  - Diabetes
  - Drugs
  - Paraneoplastic syndromes
  - Sarcoid
  - Leprosy
  - HIV.

- Demyelinating:
  - Multifocal motor neuropathy*
  - Multiple compression neuropathy (hypothyroidism, diabetes)
  - Hereditary neuropathy with liability to pressure palsies.

*This is a purely motor disorder and therefore does not cause a characteristic mononeuropathy in which both motor and sensory function is affected.

49b) The most likely diagnosis is **Churg–Strauss syndrome**.

The presence of mononeuritis multiplex in a patient with rash and previous sinusitis and late onset asthma is strongly suggestive of Churg–Strauss Syndrome, a systemic necrotizing vasculitis of the small and medium muscular-sized arteries, veins and venules. The lungs are frequently involved and severe asthma and peripheral eosinophilia are usually seen. Intra- and extravascular granulomas may occur. It often presents with symptoms of upper respiratory tract infection including sinusitis, and respiratory complaints may precede other signs of systemic vasculitis by decades. Rash, gastrointestinal and cardiac involvement is seen but the kidneys are less frequently affected than in polyarteritis nodosa, a related form of necrotizing vasculitis, in which arteries only are affected and in which the lungs are not involved. In contrast to polyarteritis nodosa, Churg–Strauss is more common in women.

49c) FBC to look for eosinophilia, CXR, ANCA, nerve biopsy

There is usually a moderate ($<20 \times 10^9$/L, >10% of the white cell count) peripheral eosinophilia (i.e. greater than that seen in atopic asthma but less than in the hypereosinophilic syndrome). CXR may show transient pulmonary infiltrates and hilar lymphadenopathy, pleural effusion, and fine and large-non cavitating nodules have been described. Tissue biopsy samples (e.g. nerve, gut) show eosinophilic infiltrates and characteristic leucocytoclastic angiitis. In some patients, antineutrophil cytoplasmic antibody (ANCA) with specificity for myeloperoxidase is found.

49d) The systemic necrotizing vasculitides (Churg–Strauss, polyarteritis nodosa and microscopic polyangiitis) all affect the nervous system and although the different subtypes have different clinical features of systemic involvement, the neurological features are similar. The majority of patients have nervous system involvement and peripheral nerve damage is nearly universal. CNS symptoms tend to occur later in the course of the disease.

Central nervous system manifestations of systemic necrotizing vasculitis may be global, with encephalopathy and seizures, or focal. Global cognitive decline is common and hallucinations and psychiatric disorders including depression, mania and paranoid psychosis may occur. Headache is common and may be related to sinusitis or aseptic meningitis. Focal abnormalities include ischaemic and haemorrhagic stroke and subarachnoid haemorrhage. Stroke may be related to hypertension, corticosteroid use or to vasculitic occlusion. Lacunar strokes affecting the basal ganglia (chorea and parkinsonism may occur) and internal capsule seem to be most common stroke subtype.

About 2% of patients have evidence of spinal cord involvement. Myelopathy may also result from cord compression from extramedullary haematoma resulting from rupture of arteritic spinal aneurysms. Vasculitic neuropathy is seen in up to 60% of patients of which mononeuritis multiplex is most common. Cranial neuropathy may occur. Involvement of several different nerves leads to confluent mononeuritis in which there is an asymmetric neuropathy affecting all four limbs. Distal symmetric polyneuropathy and cutaneous neuropathy (patchy loss of sensation over the fingers or feet) are seen but brachial plexopathy, radiculopathy and cauda equina syndrome are rare.

Neuroimaging studies in systemic nectrotizing vasculitis may be normal or show focal or multifocal infarction or haemorrhage. CSF is often normal or may show elevated pressure, increased protein and lymphocytic pleocytosis when aseptic meningitis is present. Nerve conduction studies show sensorimotor axonal neuropathy. Pathological studies of the brain show multiple areas of infarction of varying ages and inflammation of arteries and arterioles. Sural nerve biopsy shows vasculitis of the small epineural blood vessels and nerve bundle infarction may be seen.

49e) Untreated disease has a 5 year survival rate of 10%, which is improved to over 50% with steroids. Additional immunosuppressive therapy is often given particularly where there is renal, cardiac, gut or neurological involvement.

Further reading

Gross WL (2002). Churg–Strauss syndrome: update on recent developments. *Curr Opin Rheumatol*; **14**(1):11–14.

Jenette JC, Falk RJ (1997). Small vessel vasculitis. *NEJM*; **337**:1512–1523.

Noth I, Strek ME, Leff AR (2003). Churg-Strauss syndrome. *Lancet*; **361**(9370):1746.

Sehgal M, Swanson JW, Deremee RA, Colby TV (1995). Neurologic manifestations of Churg–Strauss syndrome. *Mayo Clin Proc*; **70**:337–341.

Seo P, Stone JH (2004). The antineutrophil cytoplasmic antibody-associated vasculitides. *Am J Med*; **117**(1):39–50.

Case 50

A 62-year-old woman complained of frontal headache, nausea and vomiting which had started gradually 10 days earlier. On the day of admission, she became confused and had two generalized motor seizures. She had cancer of the breast, treated with mastectomy and chemotherapy. Her last dose of chemotherapy had been 3 months previously. There was a past history of depression.

On examination, she was agitated and confused, thin and pale, with a temperature 35.9°C, pulse of 110/min and BP of 170/90 mm Hg. There was mild diffuse tenderness of the abdomen but the rest of the examination was normal.

Investigations showed:

- WCC 14.4×10^9/L (neutrophils 13.2×10^9/L).
- Na 117mmol//l, K 2.6mmol/L, glucose 8.4mmol/L, Ca 2.1mmol/L, Mg 0.3mmol/L, Alk Phos 243IU/L.
- ESR 11mm/h, CRP 12mg/L.
- CT head is shown in Fig. 50.1.
- LP: opening pressure 25cm H_2O, 24mm^3 white cells (70% mononuclear cells), 70mm^3 red cells, protein 2.9g/L, glucose 1.9mmol/L, no organisms.

Questions

50a) List the causes of seizures related to systemic cancer. Which of these are most likely in this patient?

50b) What is the abnormality on the CT scan and how would you investigate this further?

50c) Give 4 possible causes for her headache.

50d) An organism was grown following biopsy of the CT abnormality. What is the likely organism and what is the diagnosis that you would be particularly concerned about, given the clinical findings in this case? What is the treatment?

50e) Give 3 causes for the low sodium. Which of the other metabolic abnormalities exacerbates hyponatraemia?

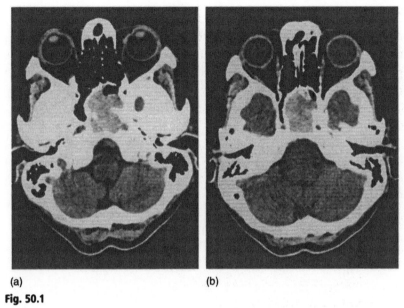

(a)   (b)

Fig. 50.1

Answers

50a) Possible causes of seizures associated with systemic malignancy include:

- Direct tumour effects:
  - Focal CNS metastasis
  - Malignant meningitis.
- Indirect tumour effects:
  - Paraneoplastic encephalitis.
- CNS infection (opportunistic).
- Drug related:
  - Chemotherapy
  - Symptomatic treatment e.g. antibiotics.
- Radiotherapy.
- Metabolic derangement:
  - Gastrointestinal upset
  - Chemotherapy
  - Poor nutrition
  - Tumour effects e.g. SIADH.
- Cerebrovascular disease:
  - CVT
  - Hypercoaguable state causing thrombosis
  - Thrombosis secondary to infection e.g. aspergillosis.

The most likely causes of this patient's seizures are **metabolic derangement, CNS infection, CVT, or malignant meningitis.** The **metabolic derangement** is likely to be multifactorial (vomiting, poor oral intake, tumour effects). A **cerebral structural abnormality** must be ruled out in any patient with systemic cancer who develops seizures. Ovarian cancer rarely metastasises to the brain (this patient had no evidence of space occupying lesion) whereas such metastases are common in breast, thyroid, melanoma, lung, renal, GI, and germ cell tumours. **Malignant meningitis** is not infrequent in ovarian cancer and may cause seizures. **CVT** (see page 10) is associated with cancer and should always be considered in patients with headache and seizures, particularly where there is a past history of thrombotic disease as in this patient. **Opportunistic CNS infections** (see page 227) are common in cancer patients particularly those receiving chemotherapy. **Paraneoplastic encephalitis** (see page 252) is uncommon but is not excluded by the investigations shown above.

50b) The CT shows **sphenoid sinus infection.**

The CT scan shows extensive high density opacity of the sphenoid sinus. There is thickening of the sinus walls. The appearances are characteristic of fungal infection. Further investigation should include aspiration/biopsy of the sinus and microbiological and histopathological examination of the sinus contents.

50c) The 4 most likely causes for her headache are:

- Sinusitis
- CNS infection
- CVT
- Malignant meningitis.

50d) The likely organism is **aspergillus fumigatus** which is the most common cause of fungal sinusitis. Rhinocerebral mucormycosis is an alternative diagnosis in diabetic patients. **Invasive aspergillosis** of the CNS is thus a possibility in this patient and parenteral antifungal treatment should be given.

The histology showed the fungal hyphae of aspergillus fumigatus. Aspergillus sinus infection together with headache, seizures, confusion and pleocytic CSF with elevated protein, suggest secondary CNS infection with aspergillus. Fungal CNS infection may cause space-occupying lesions or meningitis, and there may be granulomatous infiltrates, solitary or multiple abscesses or vasculitis. CNS aspergillosis is a cause of ischaemic stroke as the fungal hyphae invade and occlude vessels.

Aspergillus fumigatus is the most common cause of fungal sinusitis, and invasive disease occurs in association with diabetes, malnutrition, cancer, and immunosuppression. Presentation is with fever, headache,

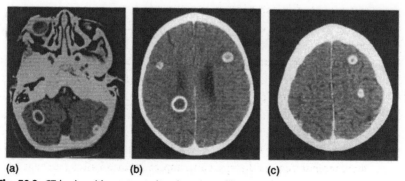

(a)　　　　　　(b)　　　　　　(c)

Fig. 50.2 CT brain with contrast showing aspergillomas.

cough, epistaxis, nasal mucosal ulceration, and eschars. Direct extension of infection may cause orbital cellulitis and associated cavernous sinus or internal carotid artery thrombosis as well as CNS infection. Examination of sinus biopsies shows fungal hyphae invading bone and blood vessels. Treatment is with surgical debridement and amphotericin B.

50e) The likely possible causes of the low sodium in this case are:

- Vomiting
- SIADH (associated with CNS pathology including malignant meningitis, CVT and opportunistic infection)
- Cerebral salt wasting (reported in association with head injury, primary brain tumours, malignant meningitis and subarachnoid haemorrhage).

Magnesium and potassium deficiency can potentiate ADH release and hence worsen hyponatraemia. The diagnosis of the cause of hyponatraemia depends on whether the patient is normovolaemic or dehydrated (see page 137). Dehydration in this case suggests vomiting or cerebral salt wasting, whereas normovolaemia suggests SIADH. In SIADH, plasma osmolarity will be low with an inappropriately concentrated urine and continued renal excretion of sodium. In vomiting with salt loss in excess of water, plasma osmolarity will be low, urine osmolarity will be high, and renal excretion of sodium will be minimal (< 10 mmol/L). Cerebral salt wasting will show low plasma osmolarity with normal urine osmolarity and inappropriately high renal sodium excretion. Treatment of cerebral salt wasting consists of water and salt supplementation in contrast to SIADH, which requires fluid restriction.

Post-mortem on this patient showed opacification of the meninges with obscuration of the roots of the lower cranial nerves, particularly the VII and VIII, and of part of the basilar artery. There was green mucinous material in the sphenoid sinus consistent with fungal sinusitis.

Further reading

Cunha BA (2001). Central nervous system infections in the compromised host: a diagnostic approach. *Infect Dis Clin North Am*; 15(2):567–590.

DeLone DR, Goldstein RA, Petermann G. *et al* (1999). Disseminated aspergillosis involving the brain: distribution and imaging characteristics. *AJNR Am J Neuroradiol*; 20(9):1597–1604.

DeShazo RD, Chapin K, Swain RE (1997). Fungal sinusitis. *Current Concepts*; 254–259.

Harrigan M (1996). Cerebral salt wasting: a review. *Neurosurgery*; 38:152.

Pruitt AA (2003). Nervous system infections in patients with cancer. *Neurol Clin*; 21(1):193–219.

Schwartz S and Thiel E (2004). Update on the treatment of cerebral aspergillosis. *Ann Hematol*; 83 Suppl 1:S42–44.

Case 51

A 78-year-old man was transferred to a tertiary referral centre with acute coronary syndrome. Shortly after transfer he became unwell and developed ST elevation consistent with full thickness myocardial infarction. He was given thrombolysis with streptokinase during which she became bradycardic and hypotensive. This resolved spontaneously but afterwards he appeared confused.

Approximately 7 hours after admission, it was noted that the patient was unable to open his eyes. He was alert and able to follow commands, and speech was normal. On examination, there was bilateral complete ptosis. The pupillary light reflex was absent bilaterally and there was bitemporal hemianopia. Eye movements were absent, as was the vestibulo-ocular reflex. Corneal reflex was intact and the remaining cranial nerves and limb examination was normal. A cranial CT and MRI were performed (see Fig. 51.1).

Questions

51a) What is the abnormality seen on the neuroimaging?

51b) What is the diagnosis? Explain the neurological findings.

51c) What is the most common cause of this syndrome?

51d) What non-neurological complications might you expect, and what further tests should you perform?

51e) How would you treat this patient?

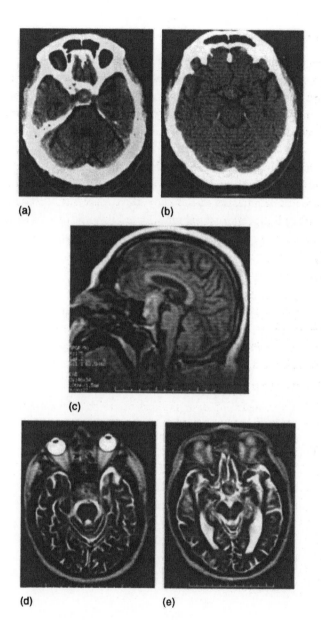

(a) (b)

(c)

(d) (e)

Fig. 51.1

Answers

51a) The neuroimaging demonstrates a **pituitary mass**.

The CT shows a pituitary mass with haemorrhage within it. The MRI shows a pituitary macroadenoma with suprasellar extension into the floor of the third ventricle, compressing the mamillary bodies. There is acute haemorrhage within the pituitary together with a low-density central lesion. The optic chiasm is involved. The tumour extends into both cavernous sinuses and possibly into the sphenoid sinuses.

51b) The diagnosis is **pituitary apoplexy** (pituitary haemorrhage or infarction).

The cardinal features of pituitary apoplexy are headache and visual loss (reduced visual acuity and/or bitemporal field loss which occur in over half of patients), variably accompanied by nausea, vomiting, opthalmoplegia, confusion, and meningism. Onset is usually acute and may mimic subarachnoid haemorrhage or meningitis but indolent progression is increasingly recognized.

In this patient, pituitary apoplexy was associated with haemorrhagic infarction of a pituitary macroadenoma caused by hypotension and streptokinase administration. Compression of the central part of the optic chiasm causes bitemporal hemianopia since the medial part of each optic nerve carries information from the nasal retina and hence the temporal visual fields. The cranial nerve signs in the case described above indicate bilateral III, IV, and VI nerve palsies. The sudden appearance of abnormalities in all these cranial nerves suggests haemorrhage into the tumour causing it to expand laterally: the III, IV, and VI nerves run lateral to the optic chiasm on their way to the cavernous sinus.

51c) Pituitary apoplexy occurs most commonly with adenomas, which may have been unrecognized previously. It may occur without obvious precipitants or in association with anticoagulation/thrombolysis, trauma, thrombocytopaenia, or diagnostic testing for pituitary adenoma e.g. dynamic hormone testing or bromocriptene therapy. Ischaemic pituitary necrosis resulting from postpartum hypotension is termed Sheehan's syndrome.

51d) Acute adrenal insufficiency develops in two thirds of patients and can be fatal. Hypogonadism, hyperprolactinaemia and GH deficiency are common and hypothyroidism may occur. Diabetes insipidus is rare. Tests should be performed for serum and urine osmolalities, and anterior pituitary hormone levels. In this patient, prolactin was 20mu/L (low), cortisol 421nmol/L (normal), TSH 0.21mu/L (normal range 0.5–5.0mu/L), testosterone 1.5nmol/L. Urine output was >200mL per hour with high normal plasma osmolality, and dilute urine consistent with diabetes insipidus.

51e) Owing to the high frequency of adrenal insufficiency, all patients should receive empirical corticosteroid treatment. This patient also required aggressive fluid resuscitation and DDAVP to treat his diabetes insipidus. Urgent neurosurgical decompression in patients with reduced level of consciousness or visual loss is generally advised (after appropriate rescusitation and steroid administration), since it is thought to improve outcome, particularly in visual impairment, and may ameliorate endocrine dysfunction. Once the acute illness has stabilized, patients should be monitored and treated for hormone deficiency.

Further reading

Chanson P, Lepeintre JF, Ducreux D (2004). Management of pituitary apoplexy. *Expert Opin Pharmacother*; 5(6):1287–1298.

Levy A (2004). Pituitary disease: presentation, diagnosis and management. *J Neurol Neurosurg Psychiatry*; 75 Suppl 3–iii47–52.

Wakai S, Fukushima T, Teramoto A, Sano K (1981). Pituitary apoplexy: its incidence and clinical significance. *J Neurosurg*; 55(2):187–193.

List of cases by clinical features at presentation (case number in italics)

Headache *1, 2, 7, 9, 22, 24, 32, 33, 34, 37, 39, 41, 43, 50*

Encephalopathy *1–3, 6, 8, 9, 11, 12, 14, 16, 17, 20, 26, 29, 30–35, 40, 41–43, 45*

Stroke/stroke-like *5, 12, 16, 17, 19, 22, 23, 25, 29*

Seizures *2, 5, 7, 16, 17, 30, 31, 50*

Weak legs *4, 18, 28, 32, 47*

Cranial neuropathy *13, 15, 21, 37, 46, 48, 51*

Peripheral neuropathy *6, 13, 15, 44, 45, 49*

Myopathy *4, 6, 18*

Movement disorder *3, 5, 8, 10, 16, 26, 27, 35, 38, 44*

List of cases by aetiological mechanism

Infectious disease *1, 7, 9, 14, 15, 21, 22, 25, 32, 35, 38, 39, 40, 43, 44, 48, 50*

Malignancy *2, 41, 42, 47*

Vascular abnormality *2, 5, 10, 12, 19, 22, 24, 27, 29, 32, 47, 51*

Endocrine/metabolic/toxic mechanism *3, 6, 8, 11, 17, 18, 20, 23, 30, 45*

Inflammatory disease *4, 16, 29, 46, 49*

Inherited conditions *17, 36*

List of cases by diagnosis

1) Herpes simplex encephalitis

2) Cerebral venous thrombosis

3) Wernicke-Korsakoff's encephalopathy

4) Dermatomyositis

5) Lateral medullary infarction

6) Hypothyroidism

7) Cryptococcus meningitis

8) Mercury poisoning

9) TB meningitis

10) Low flow TIA

11) Porphyria

12) CADASIL

13) Guillain–Barré syndrome secondary to EBV infection

14) PML and HIV infection

15) Lyme disease

16) Hashimoto's encephalopathy

17) MELAS

18) Simvastatin-associated myopathy

19) Cerebral arterial dissection

20) Thyrotoxic storm

21) Gradenigo's syndrome

22) Lemierre's syndrome

23) Hyponatraemia and stroke-like episode

24) Angiogram negative subarachnoid haemorrhage

25) Infective endocarditis

26) Malignant catatonia

27) Cerebellar haemorrhage

28) Epidural abscess

29) Isolated CNS vasculitis

30) Psychogenic polydipsia

31) Non convulsive status epilepticus

32) Meningitis and anterior spinal syndrome

33) Low pressure headache

34) Migraine coma with hemiplegia

35) New variant CJD

36) Wilson's disease

37) Idiopathic intracranial hypertension

38) Post-kidney transplant infection/lymphoma

39) Herpes simplex type 2 meningitis

40) Staphylococcal septicaemia/meningitis/hydrocephalus

41) Melanoma metastasis

42) Paraneoplastic drowsiness

43) Subdural empyema

44) HIV seroconversion and dorsal root ganglioneuronopathy

45) B12 deficiency

46) III nerve palsy and diabetes insipidus

47) Spinal cord compression/cauda equina syndrome

48) Ramsay Hunt syndrome

49) Churg–Strauss syndrome

50) Aspergillus sinusitis and CNS infection post chemotherapy

51) Pituitary apoplexy